AF731036

Biopharmaceutical Process Validation

Strategies for Risks Assessments in Real-World Applications

By

Naveenganesh Muralidharan

Published by Book Writing Pioneer
Cover design by Book Writing Pioneer
ISBN: Printed in the United States.

BOOK WRITING PIONEER

Table of Content

Dedication

To my dearest Adhvay and Adhvika,

You are the heart of my world, my greatest inspiration, and my unwavering source of joy. Every word in this book is a reflection of the lessons I hope to pass on to you—lessons of resilience, passion, and the endless pursuit of knowledge. May you always dream boldly, believe in yourselves, and know that you are capable of achieving greatness.

To my beloved father, Muralidharan, and mother, Swarnavalli,

Your love, sacrifices, and unwavering support have shaped me into the person I am today. Dad, your strength have been my guiding light, teaching me the value of perseverance and integrity. Mom, your kindness and boundless love have instilled in me the courage to chase my dreams. This book is a tribute to the foundation you built, the values you instilled, and the endless encouragement you have given me.

With all my love and gratitude,

Acknowledgment

Dear Jason Bishop and Mark Davis,

As I write this book, I want to take a moment to express my deepest gratitude to both of you.

Jason, your leadership has been truly inspiring. You have not only empowered me but have also instilled confidence in me at every step. Among the many leaders I've worked with over the past 18 years, you stand out as one of the finest people managers I have ever met. Your ability to support, guide, and bring out the best in those around you is remarkable, and I am grateful for the impact you've had on my journey.

Mark, your technical guidance and the wealth of regulatory knowledge you've shared have been invaluable. Your decades of experience have not only helped shape my understanding but have also deepened my appreciation for the complexities of this industry. Your willingness to mentor, share insights, and challenge perspectives has played a crucial role in my professional growth, and for that, I am truly thankful.

This book is, in many ways, a reflection of the knowledge, experiences, and support I've received from incredible individuals like you both. I deeply appreciate your encouragement and the role you've played in making this possible.

Chapter 1: Comprehensive Guidance on Matrix and Bracketing Validation Approaches for Microbial Control Hold Time Assessments in Biopharmaceuticals

1 Introduction

In biopharmaceutical manufacturing, maintaining product safety, consistency, and efficacy is paramount. Microbial hold time plays a critical role in ensuring these qualities throughout the production process. As regulatory agencies such as the FDA impose stringent validation requirements, it is essential to adopt robust methodologies that adequately assess microbial risks associated with hold times. This paper focuses on microbial hold time validation, specifically exploring the use of bracketing and matrix approaches to ensure a comprehensive evaluation. By addressing key parameters such as nutrient composition, hold time duration, and growth-promoting conditions, the paper offers insights into developing more reliable process validation strategies.

To facilitate this evaluation, the Cardinal microbial growth model is employed to assess growth-promoting conditions, including pH, temperature, and osmolarity, under different process scenarios. The model provides a scientific basis for understanding the potential risks associated with microbial proliferation during hold times. The paper also introduces a risk assessment framework that utilizes objective scoring matrices, which are developed as a function of mixing hydrodynamics, nutrient conditions, and the specific hold time characteristics of each process. By integrating these factors into the validation approach, this paper presents a more precise and data-driven method for evaluating microbial risks, ensuring that biopharmaceutical processes remain compliant with regulatory standards while maintaining high product quality.

2 Microbial Hold Time Studies in Biopharmaceutical Process Validation

In biopharmaceutical process validation, microbial hold time studies are critical for ensuring the quality and sterility of pharmaceutical products. These studies evaluate the stability of solutions over time, particularly their susceptibility to microbial contamination. The primary objective is to ascertain the duration for which a solution can remain in a tank, bioreactor, or other container without significant microbial growth. This information is essential for maintaining product sterility during manufacturing and preventing contamination during storage or processing delays [1].

Microbial control hold time validation establishes time limits for how long intermediate or bulk solutions can be held before further processing steps, such as filtration or sterilization. By understanding microbial risks, manufacturers can implement effective control measures to safeguard product integrity. This is particularly important to ensure that no harmful levels of bioburden compromise the product's safety before it reaches patients. The validation process involves rigorous testing and monitoring to ensure that microbial contamination does not occur, which is vital for compliance with regulatory standards and for maintaining patient safety throughout the product's lifecycle [2]. Overall, microbial hold time studies provide a comprehensive understanding of the contamination risks associated with time delays in biopharmaceutical processes. Proper validation of hold times is crucial for maintaining sterility, complying with regulatory standards, and ensuring patient safety across the product's lifecycle [1,2].

3 Setting Acceptance Criteria

3.1 Establishing Acceptance Criteria for Microbial Control Samples.

Managing hold times is crucial for microbial control and product integrity across production stages. These storage intervals between processing steps must be rigorously defined and validated based on risk assessments, with tailored strategies to address unique microbial risks. Both bioburden and endotoxin limits are initially more relaxed during early production stages to accommodate expected microbial loads. As the process advances, these limits are tightened to align with regulatory guidelines, ensuring patient safety and product quality.

3.1.1 Practices for Microbial Hold Time Management in Biopharmaceutical Production

Hold Time: Establishing acceptance criteria for microbial control during hold times is essential for maintaining product safety and integrity throughout various production stages. Hold times, defined as storage periods between processing steps, must be carefully managed to prevent microbial contamination. Each stage, from fermentation to final formulation, presents unique risks that necessitate validated hold times based on comprehensive risk assessments. For early stages, such as cell culture harvest using depth filters or a combination of centrifugation followed by depth filtration, processing typically occurs within 5 to 6 hours [3]. Muralidharan et al. (2024) demonstrated that a 12-hour pre-filtration hold time for nutrient-rich media is feasible for cell-free harvest broth from bioreactors, supported by robust microbial control strategies to prevent bioburden increases. [1]. As the process advances to intermediate stages like clarified harvest and chromatography, hold times are generally reduced to 12-24 hours to minimize microbial growth and maintain product quality [4]. In later downstream purification steps, especially before sterile filtration, hold times are often limited to 6-12 hours due to the heightened risk of contamination [5].

Managing microbial hold time for growth-promoting cell culture media and downstream buffers before sterile filtration is a critical aspect of ensuring process integrity and product safety. For cell culture media, which are designed to support cell growth, industry practices generally recommend a microbial hold time of ≤12 hours before filtration [1]. This timeframe balances sterility assurance with practical processing considerations. Similarly, for downstream buffers, microbial hold time before filtration is typically assessed within the same ≤24-hour window to confirm that they do not support microbial growth during this period [4]. Validation and adherence to these practices are essential for upholding the efficacy and safety of both cell culture media and downstream buffers.

Bioburden and endotoxin: Bioburden and endotoxin limits are crucial for maintaining microbial control throughout biopharmaceutical production. In the early upstream stages of sterile cell culture operations, bioburden limits are typically set at not more than 1 CFU/10 mL, with endotoxin limits at 10 EU/mL [1] to prevent contamination. As the process advances to intermediate stages, such as clarified harvest and product capture chromatography, bioburden limits increase to 100 CFU/10 mL but are gradually reduced to 30 and 10 CFU/10 mL as the process nears the final concentration and drug substance (DS) stage. Similarly, endotoxin limits decrease from 5 EU/mL to as low as 1 EU/mL, depending on proximity to the DS stage [6]. In the final stages of purification, prior to sterile filtration, bioburden limits are tightened to below 10 CFU/100 mL and to less than 1 CFU/10 mL in the final product. Endotoxin limits are further reduced to between 1.00 and 0.25 EU/mL [7], ensuring effective sterilization and product safety. For non-sterile products, including drug substances and drug products prior to sterile filtration, a bioburden limit of < 10 CFU/100 mL is generally considered acceptable by regulatory agencies such as the FDA and EMA, provided it is justified through process validation [8].

4 Matrix and Bracketing Approaches in Biopharmaceutical Process Validation

The matrix and bracketing approaches in process validation are strategies used to reduce the number of validation tests while ensuring comprehensive process understanding. The matrix approach involves testing a subset of variable combinations, such as different product compositions, batch sizes, or equipment settings, assuming that untested combinations will behave similarly to the tested ones. Conversely, the bracketing approach focuses on testing only the extremes of these variables—such as the smallest and largest batch sizes or highest and lowest risk conditions—assuming that the extremes will cover intermediate conditions. While a matrix allows more flexibility and broader coverage across varying conditions, bracketing is more efficient when the process behaves predictably between extreme points [9, 10].

5 Matrix and Bracketing Approaches in Microbial Hold Time And Mixing Time Validation

In microbial hold time validation, both the matrix and bracketing approaches are commonly employed to optimize the validation process while ensuring effective microbial control. The matrix approach involves testing a subset of conditions across different variables, such as solution type, storage temperature, and hold time, rather than testing every possible combination under the assumption that untested combinations will behave similarly [44]. In contrast, the bracketing approach focuses on validating the extremes of key variables, with the assumption that these extremes will adequately cover intermediate conditions.

5.1 Addressing Regulatory Concerns in Implementing Matrix / Bracketing Approach.

The use of matrix and bracketing approaches in process validation presents several risks, primarily associated with the potential for incomplete evaluation of critical process variables. These methods, while reducing the number of validation studies, may not fully capture all key variations if the grouping of products or conditions is not supported by scientific justification. As a result, gaps in data may arise, leading to insufficient evidence to ensure product consistency and safety across operational conditions. Additionally, worst-case scenarios may be underestimated, limiting the understanding of interactions between critical parameters. If not carefully implemented, product failures or quality deviations during commercial manufacturing could occur. To mitigate these risks, thorough risk assessments and scientific rationale must be applied to support the grouping strategy [10].

5.2 Preliminary Assessment and Grouping Criteria for Microbial Hold Time Validation.

Before applying the matrix or grouping approach in microbial hold time studies, it is crucial first to assess key preliminary categorical items. Establishing criteria for grouping conditions in the matrix or bracketing approach requires meeting these categorical attributes, which are summarized in Table 1. These criteria ensure that conditions within each group are effectively comparable across preparation tanks, enabling a robust process validation.

Table 1 Preliminary Categorical Attributes for Grouping Conditions in Microbial Hold Time Validation

Criterion	Description	Purpose
Material Dispensing Location	Materials dispensed from the same or similar locations.	Dispensing methods and locations can influence contamination risks and should be consistent across tanks to ensure comparability of microbial control study.
Method of Raw Material Introduction	Same or similar methods for introducing raw materials.	The method of introduction can impact the potential for microbial contamination and is essential for consistent validation results.
WFI Source	Same source of WFI or equivalent quality.	The quality of WFI can affect microbial growth and contamination risk; using the same source ensures consistency.
Cleaning and Sanitization Procedures	Same cleaning and sanitization procedures are used for raw material dispensing containers.	Variations in cleaning and sanitization methods can impact microbial contamination risks and should be consistent across tanks.
Raw material storage Conditions (Humidity / Temperature and clean room classification	Same or similar environmental conditions, including temperature and humidity.	Environmental conditions can affect microbial growth rates and hold times.
Operational Procedures	Consistent operational procedures, including filling and handling.	Variations in operational procedures can influence contamination risks and microbial behavior.

5.3 Understanding The Major Limitations of Matrix Approach And Comprehensive Risk-Based Approach.

In microbial controls hold time validation, all tanks used in the manufacturing process must be tested under at least one condition to assess potential risks. This approach is consistent with regulatory guidelines from the FDA and EMA [11, 12]. To mitigate this risk, each tank used in the manufacturing process should be tested under at least one condition to assess microbial risks.

To identify the worst-case condition from grouped conditions in a matrix approach, one should focus on the mixing hydrodynamics within the tank, as mixing and oxygenation have been shown to influence microbial growth [13]. Additionally, the matrix approach must also account for growth-promoting solution properties such as pH, temperature, osmolarity, and hold time, in combination with mixing hydrodynamics, when determining the worst-case scenario. Therefore, a comprehensive, risk-based, and quantifiable approach should be employed to thoroughly evaluate these factors, ensuring effective grouping of conditions and identification of the worst-case scenario. This approach involves the following steps:

1. *Identify All Tanks*: List all tanks used throughout the manufacturing process.

2. *Group Solutions by Tank*: Organize the solutions prepared in each tank based on Tank ID. Each solution preparation within the tanks is referred to as a "condition" within the group.

3. *Conduct a Comprehensive Risk Assessment:* Perform a detailed risk evaluation for each condition within a group to identify the worst-case scenario, focusing on microbial hold time or mixing time. This assessment is done in three stages:

1. *Evaluate Mixing Hydrodynamics:* Analyze the mixing dynamics for the grouped conditions and assign a risk score in relation to microbial control hold time and mixing time.

2. *Assess Solution Properties:* Evaluate the intrinsic properties of each solution and assign a risk score:

- For *microbial hold time*, assess factors like pH, osmolarity, temperature, hold time, and nutrient composition.

3. *Calculate Overall Risk:* Derive the overall risk score by combining the two factors (*Risk from Mixing Hydrodynamics)* × *(Risk from solution nutritional content)* × *(Risk from Solution preparation/storage conditions)*, with relevance to microbial hold time.

4. *Test Critical Conditions*: Validate the most critical conditions to ensure that microbial risks and mixing performance are effectively controlled across all tank sizes and configurations.

This method ensures a structured and thorough evaluation, enabling the identification of worst-case scenarios and maintaining control over microbial growth and mixing efficiency throughout the process.

6 Assess the mixing hydrodynamics for the grouped conditions and score the risk relevant to microbial control hold time and mixing time

In the matrix approach, for microbial validation, it is crucial to assess the variability in mixing hydrodynamics that arises from differences in mixing conditions within a group, such as variations in preparation volume, mixing speed, viscosity, and density. These differences affect the aspect ratio of the tank, which subsequently impacts critical factors such as average shear, vortex formation, air-liquid interface mass transfer rates, and overall mixing tank blend time. Therefore, a comprehensive, risk-based, and quantifiable approach should be employed to thoroughly evaluate these factors, ensuring effective grouping of conditions and identification of the worst-case scenario. This approach involves the following steps:

1. *Identify and calculate normalized engineering parameters* to assess mixing dynamics across different operating conditions and scales of operation.

2. *Assign weightage* to each normalized engineering parameter according to its influence on mixing and microbial growth.

3. *Consolidate the risk scores and weightage* for each parameter and condition assessed to compare the risks for each condition comprehensively.

6.1 Identifying normalized engineering parameters to assess mixing dynamics

Key parameters used to assess mixing performance and mass transfer efficiency in stirred tank bioreactors. These parameters, such as Power per Volume (P/V), Froude Number (Fr), and blend Time (t_{blend}) play a critical role in ensuring optimal microbial growth and mixing dynamics.

Average Shear Assessment Using Power per Volume (P/V): The P/V ratio is a crucial metric for assessing average shear across the entire preparation volume. It normalizes the effects of different impeller types, numbers, and configurations, facilitating consistent comparisons across tanks. The P/V is calculated using Eq (1) [14, 15].

$$\frac{P}{V} = \frac{N_p . \rho . N^3 . D_i^5}{V} \qquad \text{Eq (1)}$$

Vortex Formation Assessment Using Froude Number (Fr): The Froude number evaluates vortex formation by comparing inertial and gravitational forces, as shown in Eq (2) [14, 15]. In non-sparged stirred tank systems, the air-liquid interface mass transfer is influenced by the depth of the vortex and the turbulence created by the impeller. Therefore, the Froude number is used as a surrogate measure for surface mass transfer.

$$Fr = \frac{N^2 . D_i}{g} \qquad \text{Eq (2)}$$

Here, N is the impeller rotational speed, D is the impeller diameter, and g is the acceleration due to gravity (9.81 m/s^2).

Blend Time in Impeller-Agitated Systems: Differences in impeller design, scale, H/D ratio, and impeller speed significantly impact discharge rate per unit volume and overall mixing efficiency. These variations can be normalized across scales using *blend time*, which measures the time to achieve homogeneity in the tank, allowing for consistent comparison of impeller performance during scale-up or scale-down [14]. The impeller discharge rate (Q_{imp}) is calculated using the impeller flow number (N_F), agitation rate (N), and impeller diameter (di). The circulation time (t_{Cir}) is the ratio of tank volume to discharge rate, and mixing time, the time to reach 95% homogeneity, is approximately four times the circulation time [14]. Impeller flow numbers (N_F) = 0.7 to 0.9 for radial impellers and 0.3 to 0.5 [15]. Comprehensively, the mixing tank blend time can be calculated using Eq (3).

$$t_{blend} = 4 \times t_{cir} = 4 \times \left(\frac{V}{Q_{imp}}\right) = \frac{4 \times V}{N_F \times N \times d_i^3} \qquad \text{Eq (3)}$$

6.2 Assigning Weightage to Each Normalized Engineering Parameter According to its Influence on Mixing And Microbial Growth

Table 2 outlines key parameters used in assessing mixing dynamics in bioreactors, along with their assigned weightings and rationale. Each parameter's influence on processes such as turbulence, shear forces, mass transfer, and oxygen supply is considered based on its importance to the overall risk of microbial proliferation. The Height-to-Diameter (H/D) ratio is a critical factor in this evaluation, as it affects how these parameters perform in different tank configurations. The weightings reflect the relative risk significance of each parameter in controlling microbial load, with references provided to support the rationale for each assignment.

Table 2 Weightage of each normalized engineering parameter according to its influence on mixing and microbial growth

Parameter	Weight (%) Microbial Hold Time Study	Rationale for Weighting Microbial Hold Time Study
Power per Volume (P/V)	30%	High power input per unit volume enhances mixing efficiency, ensuring consistent nutrient distribution and minimizing stagnant zones where microbial growth could thrive.

Parameter	Weight (%) Microbial Hold Time Study	Rationale for Weighting Microbial Hold Time Study
Froude Number (Fr)	40%	Enhances oxygen transfer by creating vortices and waves at the gas-liquid interface, supporting microbial growth conditions.
Blend Time (t_{blend})	30%	Prolonged mixing times can elevate the likelihood of microbial contamination due to extended exposure.

6.4 Final Risk Score Calculation For Mixing Hydrodynamics

The consolidated risk score for microbial control from mixing hydrodynamics for each condition will be a weighted average of the individual risk scores for each condition within a group expressed as shown in Eq (4).

$$RS_{Mix,dynamics,i} = \left(w_{P/V} \times \frac{P/V_i}{\sum_{i=1}^{n} P/V}\right) + \left(w_{Fr} \times \frac{Fr_i}{\sum_{i=1}^{n} Fr}\right) + \left(w_{Mix,T} \times \frac{\sum_{i=1}^{n} t_{blend}}{t_{blend,i}}\right) \quad \text{Eq (4)}$$

7 Microbial Control Hold Time Testing

7.1 Assessing worst-case microbial growth promoting solution condition within a group.

Once an assessment of physical condition focusing on mixing hydrodynamics is performed, the next step is to assess the worst-case growth-promoting solution within the group. This step is essential for identifying and mitigating the highest microbial risks in the biopharmaceutical manufacturing process. The worst-case solution can be determined based on parameters like nutritional composition, preparation vessel contact surface area, pH, temperature, osmolarity, and time, which significantly influence microbial growth.

Here, risk scoring for Nutritional composition and Preparation vessel contact surface area are scored independently. However, the risk score- for growth conditions like pH, temperature, osmolarity, and time are comprehensively scored using the cardinal microbial growth model. Finally, the risk scores from mixing hydrodynamics, nutritional content and solution growth-promoting properties are consolidated together, and a comprehensive risk score is calculated.

Nutritional composition: The table below categorizes different risk levels associated with media compositions based on their potential to support microbial growth. It assigns a score to each risk level, describing the media components that contribute to this classification. This system helps in evaluating and grouping media based on their nutrient profiles and growth-promoting characteristics.

Table 3 Risk scoring guidance for grouping nutrient-rich cell culture growth media and feeds

Risk Level	Score	Description	Reference
High	5	Contains all key nutrients like carbohydrates, amino acids, vitamins, minerals, and lipids, creating an ideal environment for microbial growth.	[16, 20]
Moderate	3	Lacks carbohydrates, hormones, and serum but includes two or more essential nutrients like amino acids, vitamins, or minerals. Moderate potential for microbial growth.	
Low	1	Contains only one basic nutrient (e.g., amino acids, vitamins, minerals) with no carbohydrates or growth promotors. Low potential for microbial growth.	

Risk Level	Score	Description	Reference
No Risk	0	Contains no growth-promoting components (e.g., only salts or buffers), minimizing microbial growth risk.	

Vessel surface contact area refers to the total internal surface area of the tank that comes into contact with the solution. A larger surface area can harbor more microorganisms and provide additional sites for contamination. Thus, tanks with greater surface areas present a higher microbial risk compared to smaller tanks. The vessel surface contact area can be approximated using Eq (4). the individual risk scores for each condition within a group are expressed as shown Eq (5).

$$A_{Vessel\ Contact\ Area} = \left(\pi \times \frac{D^2}{4}\right) + (\pi . D . H) \quad \text{Eq (4)}$$

$$RS_{Vessel\ Contact\ Area} = \frac{A_{Vessel\ Contact\ Area,\ i}}{\sum_{i=1}^{n} A_{Vessel\ Contact\ Area}} \quad \text{Eq (5)}$$

7.2 Combined effects of solution conditions (temperature, pH, osmolarity and time) on microbial proliferation

The combined cardinal microbial growth model plays a crucial role in predicting microbial growth by integrating key factors like temperature, pH, and osmolarity. This model is essential for assessing microbial behavior across various conditions in biopharmaceutical process validation and quality control. By using equations developed by Rosso et al. (1995) [21], the model provides a quantitative approach to simulate how different environmental factors impact microbial proliferation, supporting effective control measures.

The Cardinal pH, Temperature, and Osmolarity Models, when combined with hold time, offer a more accurate prediction of microbial growth, helping to assess worst-case scenarios in microbial risk. This approach aids in understanding microbial dynamics under varying conditions.

As indicated by the United States Pharmacopeia (USP) <1111> "Microbiological Examination of Non-Sterile Products: Acceptance Criteria for Pharmaceutical Preparations and Substances for Pharmaceutical Use," these six microorganisms—Bacillus cereus, Bacillus subtilis, Candida albicans, Escherichia coli, Pseudomonas aeruginosa, and Staphylococcus aureus—are identified as key representatives for pharmaceutical quality assessments. A wide range of microbial populations is represented by these organisms, characterized by high resistance, spore formation, rapid growth, and pathogenicity, which are frequently encountered in pharmaceutical manufacturing environments [22]. These organisms are assessed through the cardinal model to identify worst-case growth conditions, ensuring a comprehensive microbial risk evaluation in pharmaceutical production.

Mathematical Model: The combined relative growth rate (μ_R) as a function of pH, temperature, Osmolarity and time model can be represented by Eq (6):

$$\mu_{R(T,pH,Osmo,Time)} = \frac{\mu}{\mu_{Opt}} = f(T) \times f(pH) \times f(Osmo) \times (Time) \qquad \text{Eq (6)}$$

Where μ_{opt} is the maximum growth rate under optimal conditions, and f(T), f(pH), and f(Osmo) are the individual component functions for temperature, pH, and Osmolarity, respectively.

Temperature Model f(T): The impact of temperature can be modeled using Eq (7) and Temperature cardinal growth parameters as summarized in Table 4.

$$f(T) = \begin{cases} 0 & , \quad T \leq T_{min} \; Or \; T \geq T_{max} \\ \left(\dfrac{T - T_{min}}{T_{opt} - T_{min}}\right)^{\left(\frac{T_{max}-T}{T_{max}-T_{opt}}\right)} & , \quad T_{min} \geq T \leq T_{max} \end{cases} \qquad \text{Eq (7)}$$

Table 4 Cardinal growth parameters for temperature

Microorganism	T_{min} °C	T_{opt} °C	T_{max} °C	References
Bacillus cereus	4	30-37	55	[23]
Bacillus subtilis	4	30-37	50	[24]
Candida albicans	20	37	42	[25]
Escherichia coli	7.0	37	50	[26]
Pseudomonas aeruginosa	4	37	42	[27]
Staphylococcus aureus	7.0	30-37	48	[28]

pH Model f(pH): The impact of temperature can be modeled using Eq (8) and Temperature cardinal growth parameters as summarized in Table 5.

$$f(pH) = \begin{cases} 0 & , \quad pH \leq pH_{min} \; Or \; pH \geq pH_{max} \\ \left(\frac{pH - pH_{min}}{pH_{opt} - pH_{min}}\right)^{\left(\frac{pH_{max} - pH}{pH_{max} - pH_{opt}}\right)} & , \quad pH_{min} \geq pH \leq pH_{max} \end{cases} \qquad \text{Eq (8)}$$

Table 5 Cardinal growth parameters for pH

Microorganism	pH_{min}	pH_{opt}	pH_{max}	References
Bacillus cereus	4.5	6.5	9.0	[29, 30]
Bacillus subtilis	4.5	7	9.0	[31, 32]
Candida albicans	2.5	4.0-6.5	8.0	[33]
Escherichia coli	4.0	7.0	9.0	[34]
Pseudomonas aeruginosa	5.5	7.5	9.0	[35]
Staphylococcus aureus	4.0	6.0-7.5	10	[36, 37]

Osmo Model f (Osmo): The impact of temperature can be modeled using Eq (9) and Temperature cardinal growth parameters as summarized in **Table 6** Cardinal growth parameters for osmolarity..

$$f(pH) = \begin{cases} 0, & Osmo \leq Osmo_{min}\ Or\ Osmo \geq pH_{max} \\ \dfrac{(Osmo - Osmo_{,min})(Osmo_{,max} - Osmo)}{(Osmo_{,opt} - Osmo_{,min})(Osmo_{,max} - Osmo_{,opt})}, & Osmo_{min} \geq Osmo \leq Osmo_{max} \end{cases} \quad \text{Eq (9)}$$

Table 6 Cardinal growth parameters for osmolarity

Microorganism	Osmo $_{min}$ (Osmo/Kg)	Osmo $_{Opt}$ (Osmo/Kg)	Osmo $_{Max}$ (Osmo/Kg)	References
Bacillus cereus	~0.2	~0.5 to 0.9	~1.5	[38, 39]
Bacillus subtilis	~0.2	~0.5 to 0.8	~1.2	[40, 41]
Candida albicans	~0.2	~0.6 to 0.8	~1.0	[42]
Escherichia coli	~0.1	~0.3 to 0.6	~0.9	[43, 44]
Pseudomonas aeruginosa	~0.2	~0.5 to 0.8	~1.5	[45]
Staphylococcus aureus	~0.2	~0.5 to 0.7	~1.0	[36, 37]

7.3 Comprehensive scoring for severity of microorganisms assessed

The severity of microorganisms assessed: The maximum relative growth rate of six evaluated microorganisms is used to calculate the consolidated severity score for the growth-promoting condition for each solution condition grouped, as shown in Eq (9).

$$RS_{(T,pH,Osmo,Time)} = Max\{\mu_{R(T,pH,Osmo,Time),i=BC,BS,CA,EC,PA\ and\ SA}\} \qquad \text{Eq (9)}$$

The two-letter short IDs for each microorganism are as follows:

Bacillus cereus: BC, Bacillus subtilis: BS, Candida albicans: CA, Escherichia coli: EC, Pseudomonas aeruginosa: PA, Staphylococcus aureus: SA.

7.4 Combined comprehensive risk score for microbial control hold time validation

The combined comprehensive risk score for microbial control hold time validation is calculated based on key factors, including 1. fluid mixing hydrodynamics (which considers average shear, intensity of vortex formation, and tank blend time), 2. the nutritional composition of the solution (Based on combinations of carbon source, Amino acids, growth promotors, trace elements, salts), and 3. preparation conditions (including temperature, pH, osmolarity, and preparation time). Each of these parameters plays a critical role in influencing microbial growth and contamination risk during the hold time of the process, and the overall impact on the growth is calculated from Eq (10). The weightage for parameters impacting microbial growth is summarized in Table 7.

$$\begin{aligned} RS_{Micro,Total} = {} & \left(W_{mix,Dynamics} + RS_{mix,Dynamics}\right) \\ & + \left(W_{Vessel\ Contact\ Area} + RS_{Vessel\ Contact\ Area}\right) \\ & + \left(W_{Nutrion} + RS_{Nutrition}\right) \\ & + \left(W_{T,pH,Osmo,Time} + RS_{T,pH,Osmo,Time}\right) \end{aligned} \qquad \text{Eq (10)}$$

Table 7 Weightage and Justification of Parameters Affecting Microbial Growth During Hold Time

Parameter	Weightage (%)	Justification
Mixing Dynamics	25%	Inadequate mixing can create localized pockets of poor homogenization, which may encourage microbial growth in stagnant areas. Effective mixing enhances microbial by getting oxygenation and uniform conditions.
Vessel Contact Surface Area	10%	Larger surface areas, especially rough or poorly sanitized surfaces, provide more opportunities for microbial adhesion and biofilm formation, increasing contamination risks during hold times. But often, Cleaning and sanitization processes are validated.
Nutrient Value of the Solution	35%	High nutrient content (e.g., sugars, amino acids) significantly increases the risk of microbial proliferation if microbial contamination occurs, as the media supports rapid growth.
Preparation Condition (pH, Temp, Osmolarity, Time)	30%	pH, temperature, and osmolarity conditions can dramatically impact microbial growth rates that can either promote or inhibit microbial activity. Time is a critical factor as microbial load increases with prolonged exposure.

8 Conclusion

In summary, the validation of microbial hold time is essential for maintaining the safety, consistency, and efficacy of biopharmaceutical manufacturing. This study has demonstrated the utility of the Cardinal microbial growth model in thoroughly evaluating growth-promoting conditions, including pH, temperature, osmolarity, nutrient composition, and mixing hydrodynamics. By incorporating these factors into a structured, objective scoring matrix, a more precise assessment of microbial risks and the identification of worst-case scenarios can be achieved. Furthermore, the application of bracketing and matrix approaches, combined with a comprehensive risk assessment framework, effectively addresses regulatory concerns raised by agencies such as the FDA regarding microbial hold time validation. The proposed methodology offers a data-driven and systematic approach, enhancing process validation, ensuring regulatory compliance, and ultimately supporting the production of high-quality, safe biopharmaceutical products.

References

1. Muralidharan, N., Wombaker, T., Johnson, T., & Bolduc, E. (2023, September 19). Validating prefiltration dirty-hold times for upstream media and feed solutions: Implications for establishing in-process microbial control. BioProcess International. https://www.bioprocessintl.com/sponsored-content/validating-prefiltration-dirty-hold-times-for-upstream-media-and-feed-solutions-implications-for-establishing-in-process-microbial-control
2. Sandle, T. (2015) Assessing Process Hold Times for Microbial Risks: Bioburden and Endotoxin, Journal of GXP Compliance, Vol. 19, Issue 3, Oct 2015, pp1-9
3. Bergheim, S. (2018, September 27). Choosing the best-fit cell culture harvesting technology for your process: The development of the "Mammalian Cell Culture Harvesting Guide". Biopharma Asia. https://biopharma-asia.com/magazine-articles/choosing-the-best-fit-cell-culture-harvesting-technology-for-your-process/
4. Dream, R., & Loxley, B. (2024, August 28). Process hold times: What is it and why is it important? PDA. https://www.pda.org/pda-letter-portal/home/full-article/process-hold-times-what-is-it-and-why-is-it-important
5. Hughes, P. F. (2016, January 27). Aseptic processing of biological products: Current regulatory issues. FDA/CDER/OPQ/OPF/DMA/BIV. Presented at Facing the Challenges of Drug Product and Device Development & Manufacturing, Washington, D.C. http://pmo90dc87.pic37.websiteonline.cn/upload/FDAcurrentregulatoryissues.pdf
6. Krause, S. (2015, March 16-18). Alert, action, and specification limits for bioburden and endotoxin [Conference presentation]. PDA Annual Meeting, Las Vegas, NV.
7. Yang, H., Li, N., & Chang, S. (2013). A Risk-based Approach to Setting Sterile Filtration Bioburden Limits. PDA journal of pharmaceutical science and technology, 67(6), 601–609. https://doi.org/10.5731/pdajpst.2013.00942

8. European Medicines Agency. (2019). Guideline on the sterilisation of the medicinal product, active substance, excipient and primary container (EMA/CHMP/CVMP/QWP/BWP/850374/2015). https://www.ema.europa.eu/en/documents/scientific-guideline/guideline-sterilisation-medicinal-product-active-substance-excipient-and-primary-container_en.pdf
9. Parenteral Drug Association. (2013). *Process validation: A lifecycle approach* (Technical Report No. 60). Parenteral Drug Association, Inc. https://www.pda.org/bookstore/product-detail/1931-tr-60-process-validation
10. U.S. Food and Drug Administration. (2002). Guidance for industry: Q1D bracketing and matrixing designs for stability testing of new drug substances and products. U.S. Department of Health and Human Services. https://www.fda.gov/media/71720/download
11. U.S. Food and Drug Administration. (2004). Guidance for industry: Sterile drug products produced by aseptic processing – Current good manufacturing practice. U.S. Department of Health and Human Services. https://www.fda.gov/media/71026/download
12. European Medicines Agency. (2014). Guideline on the sterilisation of the medicinal product, active substance, excipient and primary container. EMA/CHMP/CVMP/QWP/BWP/850374/2015. https://www.ema.europa.eu/en/documents/scientific-guideline/guideline-sterilisation-medicinal-product-active-substance-excipient-primary-container_en.pdf
13. Konopacki, M., Jabłońska, J., Dubrowska, K., Augustyniak, A., Grygorcewicz, B., Gliźniewicz, M., Wróblewski, E., Kordas, M., Dołęgowska, B., & Rakoczy, R. (2022). The Influence of Hydrodynamic Conditions in a Laboratory-Scale Bioreactor on Pseudomonas aeruginosa Metabolite Production. Microorganisms, 11(1), 88. https://doi.org/10.3390/microorganisms11010088
14. Doran, P. M. (2013). Bioprocess engineering principles (2nd ed.). Academic Press.
15. Benz, G. T. (2021). Agitator design for gas-liquid fermenters and bioreactors (1st ed.). Wiley.

16. Stanbury, P. F., Whitaker, A., & Hall, S. J. (2016). Principles of fermentation technology (3rd ed.). Butterworth-Heinemann.
17. Hu, W.-S. (2012). Cell culture bioprocess engineering. Springer.
18. Scientific Bio. (n.d.). A deep dive into cell culture media. Scientific Bio. Retrieved October 11, 2024, from https://www.scientificbio.com/blog/cell-culture-media.
19. Technology Networks. (n.d.). Which cell culture media is right for you? Technology Networks. Retrieved October 11, 2024, from https://www.technologynetworks.com/analysis/articles/which-cell-culture-media-is-right-for-you-352358.
20. Labome. (n.d.). Cell culture media: A review. Labome. Retrieved October 11, 2024, from https://www.labome.com/resource/Cell-Culture-Media.
21. Rosso, L., Lobry, J. R., Bajard, S., & Flandrois, J. P. (1995). Convenient Model To Describe the Combined Effects of Temperature and pH on Microbial Growth. Applied and environmental microbiology, 61(2), 610–616. https://doi.org/10.1128/aem.61.2.610-616.1995
22. United States Pharmacopeial Convention. (2020). USP <1111> Microbiological examination of non-sterile products: Acceptance criteria for pharmaceutical preparations and substances for pharmaceutical use. In USP and National Formulary (USP 43–NF 38).
23. Albaridi, N. A. (2022). Risk of bacillus cereus contamination in cooked rice. Food Science and Technology, 42. https://doi.org/10.1590/fst.108221
24. Donio, M. B. S. (2014). Antagonistic bacillus cereus tc-1 isolated from solar salt work in southern India. Journal of Microbial &Amp; Biochemical Technology, 06(05). https://doi.org/10.4172/1948-5948.1000151
25. Sardi, J. d. C. O., Scorzoni, L., Bernardi, T., Fusco-Almeida, A. M., & Mendes-Giannini, M. J. S. (2013). Candida species: current epidemiology, pathogenicity, biofilm formation, natural antifungal products and new therapeutic options. Journal of Medical Microbiology, 62(1), 10-24. https://doi.org/10.1099/jmm.0.045054-0
26. Fujikawa, H., Kai, A., & Morozumi, S. (2003). A new logistic model for bacterial growth. Journal of the Food Hygienic Society of Japan

(Shokuhin Eiseigaku Zasshi), 44(3), 155-160. https://doi.org/10.3358/shokueishi.44.155

27. Sardi, J. d. C. O., Scorzoni, L., Bernardi, T., Fusco-Almeida, A. M., & Mendes-Giannini, M. J. S. (2013). Candida species: current epidemiology, pathogenicity, biofilm formation, natural antifungal products and new therapeutic options. Journal of Medical Microbiology, 62(1), 10-24. https://doi.org/10.1099/jmm.0.045054-0
28. Kim, Y. H., Nam, G. W., & Yoon, K. S. (2018). Growth and survival of staphylococcus aureus on beef jerky as a function of temperature. Journal of Food Safety, 38(5). https://doi.org/10.1111/jfs.12495
29. Saeid, A., Prochownik, E., & Dobrowolska−Iwanek, J. (2018). Phosphorus solubilization by bacillus species. Molecules, 23(11), 2897. https://doi.org/10.3390/molecules23112897
30. Gao, T., Foulston, L., Chai, Y., Wang, Q., & Losick, R. (2015). Alternative modes of biofilm formation by plant-associated bacillus cereus. MicrobiologyOpen, 4(3), 452-464. https://doi.org/10.1002/mbo3.251
31. Chen, L., Cao, C., Wang, S., Varcoe, J. R., Slade, R. C. T., Avignone–Rossa, C., … & Zhao, F. (2019). Electron communication of bacillus subtilis in harsh environments. iScience, 12, 260-269. https://doi.org/10.1016/j.isci.2019.01.020
32. Verma, J. P., Jaiswal, D. K., Krishna, R., Prakash, S., Yadav, J., & Singh, V. (2018). Characterization and screening of thermophilic bacillus strains for developing plant growth promoting consortium from hot spring of Leh and Ladakh region of India. Frontiers in Microbiology, 9. https://doi.org/10.3389/fmicb.2018.01293
33. Sardi, J. d. C. O., Scorzoni, L., Bernardi, T., Fusco-Almeida, A. M., & Mendes-Giannini, M. J. S. (2013). Candida species: current epidemiology, pathogenicity, biofilm formation, natural antifungal products and new therapeutic options. Journal of Medical Microbiology, 62(1), 10-24. https://doi.org/10.1099/jmm.0.045054-0
34. Fujikawa, H., Kai, A., & Morozumi, S. (2003). A new logistic model for bacterial growth. Journal of the Food Hygienic Society of Japan

(Shokuhin Eiseigaku Zasshi), 44(3), 155-160. https://doi.org/10.3358/shokueishi.44.155

35. Sardi, J. d. C. O., Scorzoni, L., Bernardi, T., Fusco-Almeida, A. M., & Mendes-Giannini, M. J. S. (2013). Candida species: current epidemiology, pathogenicity, biofilm formation, natural antifungal products and new therapeutic options. Journal of Medical Microbiology, 62(1), 10-24. https://doi.org/10.1099/jmm.0.045054-0
36. Tango, C. N., Akkermans, S., Hussain, M. S., Khan, I., Impe, J. V., Jin, Y., … & Oh, D. H. (2018). Modeling the effect of pH, water activity, and ethanol concentration on biofilm formation of Staphylococcus aureus. Food Microbiology, 76, 287-295. https://doi.org/10.1016/j.fm.2018.06.006
37. Iyer, V., Raut, J. S., & Dasgupta, A. (2021). Impact of pH on growth of staphylococcus epidermidis and staphylococcus aureus in vitro. Journal of Medical Microbiology, 70(9). https://doi.org/10.1099/jmm.0.001421
38. Carlin, F., Albagnac, C., Rida, A., Guinebretière, M., Couvert, O., & Nguyen-Thé, C. (2013). Variation of cardinal growth parameters and growth limits according to phylogenetic affiliation in the bacillus cereus group. Consequences for risk assessment. Food Microbiology, 33(1), 69-76. https://doi.org/10.1016/j.fm.2012.08.014
39. Stiller, A., Fink, A., & Mitchell, D. J. (2020). Bacillus cereus & bacillus pumilus harvested from a copper roof inhibit the growth of other microorganisms. American Journal of Undergraduate Research, 17(2), 3-11. https://doi.org/10.33697/ajur.2020.016
40. Carlin, F., Albagnac, C., Rida, A., Guinebretière, M., Couvert, O., & Nguyen-Thé, C. (2013). Variation of cardinal growth parameters and growth limits according to phylogenetic affiliation in the bacillus cereus group. Consequences for risk assessment. Food Microbiology, 33(1), 69-76. https://doi.org/10.1016/j.fm.2012.08.014
41. Carlin, F., Albagnac, C., Rida, A., Guinebretière, M., Couvert, O., & Nguyen-Thé, C. (2013). Variation of cardinal growth parameters and growth limits according to phylogenetic affiliation in the bacillus cereus group. consequences for risk assessment. Food Microbiology, 33(1), 69-76. https://doi.org/10.1016/j.fm.2012.08.014

42. Sardi, J. d. C. O., Scorzoni, L., Bernardi, T., Fusco-Almeida, A. M., & Mendes-Giannini, M. J. S. (2013). Candida species: current epidemiology, pathogenicity, biofilm formation, natural antifungal products and new therapeutic options. Journal of Medical Microbiology, 62(1), 10-24. https://doi.org/10.1099/jmm.0.045054-0
43. Смирнова, Г. В., Muzyka, N. G., & Oktyabrsky, O. N. (2000). The role of antioxidant enzymes in response of escherichia coli to osmotic upshift. FEMS Microbiology Letters, 186(2), 209-213. https://doi.org/10.1111/j.1574-6968.2000.tb09106.x
44. Rojas, E., Theriot, J. A., & Huang, K. C. (2014). Response of escherichia coli growth rate to osmotic shock. Proceedings of the National Academy of Sciences, 111(21), 7807-7812. https://doi.org/10.1073/pnas.1402591111
45. Sardi, J. d. C. O., Scorzoni, L., Bernardi, T., Fusco-Almeida, A. M., & Mendes-Giannini, M. J. S. (2013). Candida species: current epidemiology, pathogenicity, biofilm formation, natural antifungal products and new therapeutic options. Journal of Medical Microbiology, 62(1), 10-24. https://doi.org/10.1099/jmm.0.045054-0

Chapter 2: Comprehensive Guidance on Risk Assessment for Buffer and Solution Mixing Time Validation using Matrix Approach.

1 Introduction

In biological manufacturing, the validation of mixing processes plays a vital role in ensuring product quality and regulatory compliance. As biologics are often complex multicomponent solutions, achieving consistent homogeneity in mixing is a critical parameter for successful production. Variations in mixing can lead to inconsistencies in the final product, affecting efficacy, stability, and safety. Given the increased focus of regulatory bodies on process consistency, it becomes imperative to validate mixing times comprehensively and efficiently.

One prominent approach to addressing these challenges is the matrix and bracketing method, which allows for the optimization of mixing validation across different solution formulations. This approach aims to identify and validate worst-case scenarios, streamlining the validation process while meeting regulatory requirements. However, this method must be supported by a robust, quantitative risk assessment framework that considers key factors influencing mixing effectiveness.

This paper introduces such a framework, evaluating mixing performance as a function of hydrodynamic conditions, solubility limits, particle size distribution, and the impact of chemical complexity and ionic strength. By developing this structured risk assessment strategy, the paper seeks to guide biological manufacturers in establishing a validated mixing process that aligns with regulatory standards, thereby enhancing consistency in product quality and operational efficiency.

2 Mixing time studies in biopharmaceutical process validation

In biopharmaceutical process validation, manufacturers conduct mixing time studies to ensure consistent product formulation throughout the manufacturing process. These studies determine the time needed to achieve a homogeneous solution, which is crucial for maintaining uniform product quality and efficacy. By proactively identifying and addressing potential issues related to inadequate mixing, such as localized variations in concentration or pH, manufacturers mitigate risks and maintain consistency in product quality. Accurate mixing validation allows them to establish robust operational controls, ensuring even distribution of all ingredients and consistent achievement of critical quality attributes. Ultimately, successful mixing time validation helps manufacturers meet regulatory standards and protect product quality throughout the manufacturing lifecycle [1, 2].

3 Setting acceptance criteria

To ensure consistency and control in manufacturing, especially during process validation, it is critical to monitor key parameters that influence mixing time and overall homogeneity. Mixing time is a fundamental parameter in determining whether the process achieves a uniform distribution of components within the required time frame.

3.1 Acceptable sample size to establish homogeneity criteria

Using three consecutive samples helps confirm process stability and ensures that measured parameters remain consistently within acceptable limits, thereby strengthening the reliability of the mixing process. For normally distributed parameters, the required sample size at a given confidence, power, and detectability is calculated using Eq (11) [3].

$$n_s = \frac{\left(Z_{1-\alpha/2} + Z_{1-\beta}\right)^2}{\left(\frac{\Delta}{\sigma}\right)^2} \quad \textit{for a two sided paramter specification} \qquad \text{Eq (11)}$$

Where n_s is the sample size, and $Z_{1-\alpha}$ and $Z_{1-\beta}$ are the inverse cumulative Z values corresponding to the type I error (α) and the type II error (β). A typical α value is set at 0.05, indicating a 5% risk of falsely rejecting a true null hypothesis, leading to a confidence level of 95% [4]. For β, a common value is 0.20, implying an 80% reliability or a 20% chance of failing to reject a false null hypothesis [5]. The detectability (Δ/σ) represents the acceptable deviation from the mean, expressed in a number of standard deviations. According to

FDA guidance, a Δ/σ of 1.0 at 90% confidence and 80% reliability is sufficient to conclude that the sample represents the population [6]. Under these conditions, the calculated sample size is three, validating the use of three consecutive samples to establish process consistency.

3.2 Critical consideration for setting homogeneity acceptance criteria

To establish homogeneity, the criteria include either maintaining a relative standard deviation (RSD) of individual results within ≤ 5.0% or ensuring that all individual values remain within ±10.0% of the average [3]. When measurements are reported near the lower end of the range, absolute values are applied to validate the required precision for achieving homogeneity. The methods, along with their corresponding absolute values, frequently reported in mixing time study validations, are detailed below.

3.2.1 Acceptable variability limits are utilized to confirm homogeneity.

Monitoring at least one critical parameter related to mixing, such as turbidity, conductivity, pH, or osmolarity, is recommended to ensure the process remains within acceptable limits. While not all parameters need to be assessed in every case, it is essential to establish and rigorously monitor acceptance criteria for mixing time to verify homogeneity.

Visual confirmation, as defined by USP <790>, is employed to ensure particle-free solutions and assess mixing efficiency when detailed measurements are not feasible [4, 5].

Turbidity is controlled below 5 NTU to maintain solution clarity and verify the absence of particulate matter, indicating complete mixing [6, 7].

Conductivity is closely monitored to reflect the solution's ionic content, with deviations typically restricted to ±2 to ±3 µS/cm to ensure uniform ionic distribution and process consistency [8]. In non-critical processes, broader limits of up to ±5 µS/cm or ±5% may be utilized, offering flexibility while maintaining control [9, 9].

The pH range is typically set within ±0.03 to ±0.05 units to maintain a consistent chemical environment, thereby ensuring homogeneous conditions throughout the solution [11, 12]. In weak acid solutions, such as CO_2-bicarbonate-mediated buffers, as well as cell culture growth media and feeds, mixing time can significantly impact the solution's pH. In such cases, achieving consistent pH values across three consecutive samples to confirm solution homogeneity is often impractical. Consequently, using pH assessment within a narrow range across three samples is not recommended as a criterion for evaluating homogeneity.

Osmolarity is set within a ±5 mOsmo/Kg range to ensure homogeneity [17, 18].

4 Matrix and Bracketing Approaches in Mixing Time Studies

The matrix and bracketing approaches are essential strategies in mixing time validation for biopharmaceutical processes aimed at optimizing efforts while ensuring process consistency. The matrix approach involves testing a representative subset of variable combinations, such as batch sizes, agitator speeds, and tank geometries, to understand their impact on mixing efficiency. For example, in a bioreactor, a matrix study might assess various combinations like 100 L, 500 L, and 1000 L batches with agitator speeds of 100 RPM and 200 RPM and different tank geometries, assuming that untested conditions will behave similarly. In contrast, the bracketing approach focuses on testing the extremes of key variables, such as the smallest and largest batch sizes and the lowest and highest agitator speeds, under the assumption that intermediate conditions will perform consistently. This approach is particularly useful when the process behaves predictably between these extreme points. Both methods offer distinct advantages, allowing manufacturers to streamline validation efforts while ensuring effective mixing and maintaining control over the process.

4.1 Understanding the major limitations of matrix and bracketing approach and comprehensive risk-based approach.

In mixing time process validation, all tanks used in the manufacturing process must be tested under at least one condition to assess potential risks. This approach is consistent with regulatory guidelines from the FDA and EMA [19, 20]. In practice, not all preparation tanks are geometrically similar, differing in factors such as aspect ratio, impeller location, number of impellers, and impeller-to-tank diameter ratio. These variations make it challenging to demonstrate consistent mixing across different scales by solely validating extreme conditions under a bracketing approach. To address this risk, it is recommended that every tank be tested under specific conditions in mixing studies to ensure robust process validation.

To identify the worst-case condition from grouped conditions in a matrix approach, one should focus on the mixing hydrodynamics within the tank, maximum solubility of the multicomponent solution, particle size of powders used and immiscibility assessment based on chemical complexity & ionic strength [21]. Therefore, a comprehensive, risk-based, and quantifiable approach should be employed to thoroughly evaluate these factors, ensuring effective grouping of conditions and identification of the worst-case scenario. This approach involves the following steps:

5. *Identify All Tanks*: List all tanks used throughout the manufacturing process.

6. *Group Solutions by Tank*: Organize the solutions prepared in each tank based on Tank ID. Each solution preparation within the tanks is referred to as a "condition" within the group.

7. *Conduct a Comprehensive Risk Assessment:* Perform a detailed risk evaluation for each condition within a group to identify the worst-case scenario, focusing on microbial hold time or mixing time. This assessment is done in three stages:

1. *Evaluate Mixing Hydrodynamics:* Analyze the mixing dynamics for the grouped conditions and assign a risk score in relation to solution solubility.

2. *Calculate Overall Risk:* Derive the overall risk score by combining the factors: *(Risk from Mixing Hydrodynamics)* × *(Risk from solution maximum solubility)* × *(Risk from particle size)* × *(Risk from chemical complexity & ionic strength.)* as shown in Figure 1.

8. *Test Critical Conditions*: Validate the most critical conditions to ensure that microbial risks and mixing performance are effectively controlled across all tank sizes and configurations.

This method ensures a structured and thorough evaluation, enabling the identification of worst-case scenarios and maintaining control over microbial growth and mixing efficiency throughout the process.

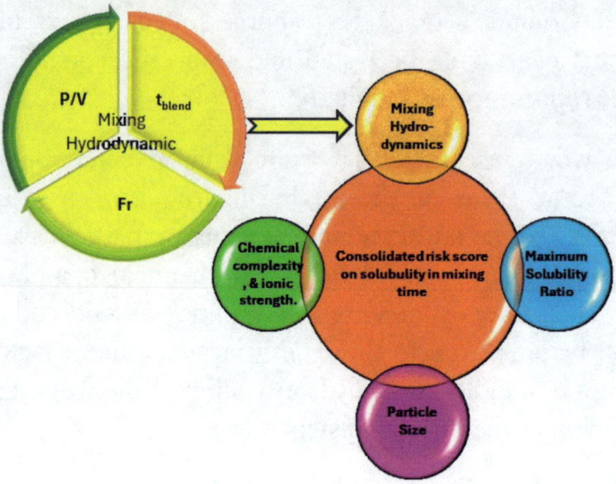

Figure 1 *Comprehensive risk assessment for buffers & solution mixing time studies using matrix approach.*

5 Mixing hydrodynamics

In the matrix approach, both for mixing and microbial validation, it is crucial to assess the variability in mixing hydrodynamics that arise from differences in mixing conditions within a group, such as variations in preparation volume, mixing speed, viscosity, and density. These differences affect the aspect ratio of the tank, which subsequently impacts critical factors such as average shear, vortex formation, air-liquid interface mass transfer rates, and overall mixing tank blend time. Therefore, a comprehensive, risk-based, and quantifiable approach should be employed to thoroughly evaluate these factors, ensuring effective grouping of conditions and identification of the worst-case scenario. This approach involves the following steps:

4. *Identify normalized engineering parameters* to assess mixing dynamics across different operating conditions and scales of operation.

5. *Assign a risk score* based on the percentage difference between the maximum and minimum within the grouped conditions.

6. *Assign weightage* to each normalized engineering parameter according to its influence on mixing and microbial growth.

7. *Consolidate the risk scores and weightage* for each parameter and condition assessed to compare the risks for each condition comprehensively.

5.1 Identifying Normalized Engineering Parameters to Assess Mixing Dynamics

Key parameters used to assess mixing performance and mass transfer efficiency in stirred tank bioreactors. These parameters, such as Power per Volume (P/V), Froude Number (Fr), and blend Time (t_{blend}), play a critical role in ensuring optimal microbial growth and mixing dynamics.

Average Shear Assessment Using Power per Volume (P/V): The P/V ratio is a crucial metric for assessing average shear across the entire preparation volume. It normalizes the effects of different impeller types, numbers, and configurations, facilitating consistent comparisons across tanks. The P/V is calculated using Eq (1) [22, 23].

$$\frac{P}{V} = \frac{N_p . \rho . N^3 . D_i^5}{V} \qquad \text{Eq (12)}$$

Vortex Formation Assessment Using Froude Number (Fr): The Froude number evaluates vortex formation by comparing inertial and gravitational forces, as shown in Eq (2) [22, 23]. In non-sparged stirred tank systems, the air-liquid interface mass transfer is influenced by the depth of the vortex and the turbulence created by the impeller. Therefore, the Froude number is used as a surrogate measure for surface mass transfer.

$$Fr = \frac{N^2 . D_i}{g} \qquad \text{Eq (13)}$$

Where N is the impeller rotational speed, D is the impeller diameter, and g is the acceleration due to gravity (9.81 m/s^2).

Blend Time in Impeller-Agitated Systems: Differences in impeller design, scale, H/D ratio, and impeller speed significantly impact discharge rate per unit volume and overall mixing efficiency. These variations can be normalized across scales using *blend time*, which measures the time to achieve homogeneity in the tank, allowing for consistent comparison of impeller performance during scale-up or scale-down [22]. The impeller discharge rate (Q_{imp}) is calculated using the impeller flow number (N_F), agitation rate (N), and impeller diameter (di). The circulation time (t_{Cir}) is the ratio of tank volume to discharge rate, and mixing time, the time to reach 95% homogeneity, is approximately four times the circulation time [22]. Impeller flow numbers (N_F) = 0.7 to 0.9 for radial impellers and 0.3 to 0.5 [23]. Comprehensively, the mixing tank blend time can be calculated using Eq (3).

$$t_{blend} = 4 \times t_{cir} = 4 \times \left(\frac{V}{Q_{imp}}\right) = \frac{4 \times V}{N_F \times N \times d_i^3}$$

5.2 Assigning Weightage To Each Normalized Engineering Parameter According To Its Influence On Mixing And Microbial Growth

Table 1 outlines key parameters used in assessing mixing dynamics in bioreactors, along with their assigned weightings and rationale. Each parameter's influence on processes such as turbulence, shear forces, mass transfer, and oxygen supply is considered based on its importance to overall mixing performance, especially in large-scale operations. The Height-to-Diameter (H/D) ratio is a critical factor in this evaluation, as it affects how these parameters perform in different tank configurations. The weightings reflect the relative significance of each parameter in ensuring efficient and uniform mixing, with references provided to support the rationale for each assignment.

Table 1 Weightage of each normalized engineering parameter according to its influence on mixing and microbial growth

Parameter	Weight (%) for Mixing Time Study	Rationale for Weighting for Mixing Time Study
Power per Volume (P/V)	30%	Crucial for energy input and turbulence, which are essential for achieving uniform mixing, particularly in large bioreactors.
Froude Number (Fr)	25%	Vortex formation helps to dissolve solid components into a solution.
Mixing Time (t_b)	30%	Indicates how long it takes to achieve homogeneity but is a secondary concern in high-energy mechanical mixing studies.

5.3 Final risk score calculation for mixing hydrodynamics

The final score will be a weighted average of the individual risk scores for each parameter, as expressed in Eq ().

$$RS_{Mix,dynamics,i} = \left(w_{P/V} \times \frac{\sum_{i=1}^{n} P/V}{P/V_i}\right) + \left(w_{Fr} \times \frac{\sum_{i=1}^{n} Fr_i}{Fr}\right) + \left(w_{Mix,T} \times \frac{t_{blend,i}}{\sum_{i=1}^{n} t_{blend}}\right)$$

The acceptable final risk score, incorporating parameters such as Power per Volume (P/V), Froude Number (Fr), Mass Transfer Coefficient (KLa), and Tank Blend Time, assesses the risk from mixing hydro dynamics within different conditions grouped.

6 Maximum Solubility Ratio

Osmolarity is defined as the measure of solute concentration per liter of solution, expressed in osmoles per liter (Osm/L). It accounts for all solute particles in the solution, including ions, molecules, and complexes [26]. Maximum solubility refers to the highest concentration of a solute that can dissolve in a solvent at a given temperature and pressure before reaching saturation. Beyond this point, additional solutes will not dissolve and may precipitate [27]. Osmolarity corresponding to the maximum solubility is termed as maximum solubility osmolarity (MSO).

Example: Consider a solution containing sodium chloride (NaCl) and glucose.

Step 1: Calculate the maximum solubility osmolarity for NaCl, Molecular weight of NaCl is MW_{NaCl}=58.44 g/mol, and maximum solubility of NaCl is C_{sat}= 357 g/L, and NaCl Sodium chloride (NaCl) dissociates into two ions (Na+) and (Cl-), so the number of particles produced n_{NaCl} =2. Therefore, maximum solubility Osmolarity of NaCl solution is calculated as shown in Eq (16).

$$MSO_{NaCl} = n \times \left(\frac{C_{Sat}\ g/L}{MW\ g/mol}\right) = 2 \times \left(\frac{357\ g/L}{58.44\ g/mol}\right) = 12.2\ Osm/L$$

Step 2: Calculate maximum solubility osmolarity for Glucose. Molecular weight of NaCl is MW_{Glc} =180.16 g/mol, and maximum solubility of Glc is C_{sat}= 1,200 g/L, and Glucose does not dissociate in water, so the number of particles produced n_{Glc} =1. Therefore, maximum solubility Osmolarity of NaCl solution is calculated as shown in Eq (17).

$$MSO_{Glc} = n \times \left(\frac{C_{Sat}\ g/L}{MW\ g/mol}\right) = 1 \times \left(\frac{1{,}200\ g/L}{180.16\ g/mol}\right) = 6.67\ Osm/L$$

Step 3: The total osmolarity is the sum of the osmolarity contributions from each solute, as shown in Eq (18).

$$MSO_{Total} = 12.2 + 6.67 = 18.87\ Osm/L$$

Maximum Solubility Ratio (MSR): In multi-component solutions, osmolarity can provide insights into the solubility behavior of the components. When the osmolarity of a solution approaches the osmolarity corresponding to the maximum solubility of one or more solutes, it indicates that the solution is nearing saturation. Therefore, the ratio of osmolarity to maximum solubility osmolarity, defined as Maximum Solubility Ratio (MSR), can serve as a useful surrogate measure of maximum solubility [28, 29]. For illustration maximum solubility ratio for a solution containing 58.44 g/L NaCl and 180.16 g/L glucose is shown in Eq (19) to Eq (21).

$$Osm_{NaCl} = n \times \left(\frac{C\ g/L}{MW\ g/mol}\right) = 2 \times \left(\frac{29.22\ g/L}{58.44\ g/mol}\right) = 1.0\ Osm/L \qquad \text{Eq (19)}$$

$$Osm_{Glc} = n \times \left(\frac{C\ g/L}{MW\ g/mol}\right) = 1 \times \left(\frac{180.16\ g/L}{180.16\ g/mol}\right) = 1.0\ Osm/L \qquad \textit{Eq (20)}$$

$$Osm_{Total} = Osm_{NaCl} + Osm_{Glc} = 2.0\ Osm/L \qquad \textit{Eq (21)}$$

$$MSR = \frac{OSm_{Total}}{MSO_{Total}} = \frac{2\ Osm/L}{18.87\ Osm/L} = 0.106 \qquad \textit{Eq (22)}$$

7 Particle Size

Buffer salts and powders are typically categorized by their particle size distribution, which substantially affects their dissolution rates and handling characteristics. Various vendors in the biopharmaceutical industry offer buffer salts and powders with specific particle size classifications to meet different dissolution and handling requirements. These products are offered in forms ranging from course to fine powders, with detailed particle size distributions provided in vendor-provided technical documentation (specification sheets, product catalogs, or technical data sheets). For risk assessment purposes, particles are classified based on USP<8111> guidelines for powder fineness [30], as shown in Table 2. When more than one powder component is added for a single solution makeup, the consolidated particle risk score CPRS for a single solution is calculated as shown in EQ. Here, ni is the number of powder components compounded in a solution makeup, and PRSi is the risk score of each component in the solution makeup.

$$CPRS = \frac{\sum PRS_i}{n_i \times 4}$$

Table 2 Risk assessment scoring for particle size

Risk Level	Score	Description
Low	1	Very fine particles are typically classified as those ranging from ≤ 125 μm.
Moderate	2	Fine particles are typically classified as those ranging from 125-180 μm.
High	3	Coarse particles are generally defined as those are 180-355 (μm).
Very High	4	Large particles (>355 μm) dissolve slowly and risk incomplete mixing.

8 Chemical Complexity and Ionic Strength.

Table 3 categorizes solutions used in biologics manufacturing based on their chemical complexity and ionic strength on dissolving risk, with scores ranging from 1 to 4. Low-risk solutions, like simple salts and buffers, dissolve easily, while moderate-risk solutions, such as amino acids and polysaccharides, may require pH adjustments or careful mixing. High-risk groups include proteins and viscous solutions that can pose challenges due to aggregation or high viscosity. Very high-risk solutions, such as complex compounds and suspensions, require specialized mixing techniques due to their poor solubility and phase separation tendencies.

Table 3 Risk assessment scoring for Chemical complexity and ionic strength.

Risk Level	**Score**	**Description**	**Examples**
Low	1	High solubility, no complex interactions, straightforward preparation, and low viscosity (< 10 cP) in typical concentrations.	Simple salts: Sodium chloride ($NaCl$), potassium chloride (KCl), magnesium sulfate ($MgSO_4$), etc. Buffers: Phosphate-buffered saline (PBS), Tris buffer, acetate buffer. Sugars: Glucose, sucrose, trehalose.
Moderate	2	Soluble, but some may require pH adjustment or have slower dissolving kinetics. Generally soluble but may have moderate mixing times based on concentration and temperature.	Amino acids: Glycine, L-glutamine, arginine. Polysaccharides: Hydroxypropyl methylcellulose (HPMC), dextran. Certain vitamins, typical cell media formulations and co-factors: Niacinamide riboflavin.

Risk Level	Score	Description	Examples
High	3	High molecular weight, potential for aggregation, and stability issues affecting dissolution and mixing times. It can be slow to dissolve, especially at higher concentrations, and can impact mixing due to foaming tendencies. High viscosity increases mixing times and requires careful handling to ensure homogeneity. It can interact with ions or proteins, requiring slow, controlled addition to prevent precipitation or instability.	Proteins: Monoclonal antibodies, bovine serum albumin (BSA), recombinant proteins. Detergents and Surfactants: Polysorbates (Tween 20/80), Triton X-100. High-concentration viscous solutions: Glycerol, polyethylene glycol (PEG). Chelators and stabilizers: EDTA, citrate, non-polar amino acids feed, and high-concentration cell culture feeds
Very High	4	Poor water solubility and tendency to form separate phases or aggregates requiring specialized mixing techniques or solvents. Require mechanical dispersion or high-shear mixing, with precise control over mixing time and speed	Complex compounds: Lipids, cholesterol, and micelle-forming agents. Suspensions and emulsions: Alum-based adjuvants, lipid nanoparticles.

9 Combined comprehensive risk score for mixing time validation.

To consolidate the various risk factors into a single comprehensive score, we employed a weighted sum formula. Each parameter—maximum solubility ratio or solution complexity, viscosity, and particle size distribution and mixing hydrodynamics—was assigned a weight based on its relative significance in determining solution stability and solubility. The comprehensive score was calculated using the Eq (24):

$$Mixing\ Risk\ Score = \sum_i (S_i \times W_i) \qquad \text{Eq (24)}$$

Where $\mathbf{S_i}$ represents the individual score, and $\mathbf{W_i}$ denotes the corresponding weighting factor for each parameter. This approach allows for a quantifiable assessment of the cumulative risk, with higher scores indicating increased risk to solubility in the system.

Table 4 Weightage of different factors impacting solubility of components in a solution

Parameters	Weightage	Reason
Mixing Hydro Dynamics	20%	While mixing, hydrodynamics primarily influences the physical mixing and dispersion of components, they do not directly alter the chemical properties and saturation limit that limit or drive solubility.
Maximum Solubility Ratio	30%	The solubility ratio determines the extent to which a component can dissolve; a higher capacity allows the system to reach equilibrium faster and more efficiently.
Particle Size	10%	Smaller particle size increases the surface area, shortening diffusion paths and enhancing dissolution, but

Parameters	Weightage	Reason
		it is weighted lower due to the dominant influence of hydrodynamics and solubility limits.
Chemical complexity and ionic strength.	40%	Chemical Complexity and Ionic Strength have a higher weightage than Maximum Solubility Ratio because they dynamically affect solubility through interactions like aggregation, bonding, and ion pairing, which significantly influence the stability and behavior of solutions at the manufacturing scale beyond maximum solubility limits that are pre- evaluated at small scale during process development.

10 Conclusion

Validation of mixing times in biological manufacturing is a crucial process for ensuring the consistency, quality, and safety of biologics. This paper highlights the importance of implementing a comprehensive approach that leverages the matrix and bracketing strategy to address regulatory challenges efficiently. By focusing on key variables such as hydrodynamics, maximum solubility, particle size distribution, and chemical complexity, manufacturers can systematically evaluate and optimize their mixing processes. The development of a quantifiable risk assessment framework allows for a deeper understanding of the factors impacting mixing outcomes, facilitating better decision-making and process control. This structured methodology not only helps in achieving regulatory compliance but also enhances product uniformity and operational efficiency. Ultimately, by adopting these strategies, manufacturers can proactively mitigate risks associated with mixing, ensure alignment with regulatory standards, and maintain high-quality production standards in biologics manufacturing. This paper serves as a guide to implementing a scientific and risk-based approach to mixing validation, supporting the continuous improvement of biomanufacturing processes.

References

1. Fulton, B., & Gorsky, I. (2024). Risk- and science-based media and buffer mixing validations. Pharmaceutical Engineering, March/April 2024. Retrieved from https://ispe.org/pharmaceutical-engineering/march-april-2024/risk-and-science-based-media-and-buffer-mixing
2. ECA Academy. (2022, June 8). Validation of mixing uniformity is also required for active ingredients. Retrieved from https://www.gmp-compliance.org/gmp-news/validation-of-mixing-uniformity-also-required-for-active-ingredients
3. NIST/SEMATECH. (2012). Handbook of Statistical Methods. NIST. https://doi.org/10.18434/M32189
4. Lakens, D. (2013). Calculating and reporting effect sizes to facilitate cumulative science: A practical primer for t-tests and ANOVAs. Frontiers in Psychology, 4, Article 863. https://doi.org/10.3389/fpsyg.2013.00863
5. Durivage, M. (2016, October 27). How to establish sample sizes for process validation using statistical tolerance intervals. Bioprocess Online. https://www.bioprocessonline.com/doc/how-to-establish-sample-sizes-for-process-validation-using-statistical-tolerance-intervals-0001
6. Weng, Y. (2016, March 21). Statistical review and evaluation. U.S. Food and Drug Administration. https://www.fda.gov/media/105013/download
7. U.S. Food and Drug Administration. (2003). Guidance for industry: Powder blends and finished dosage units — Stratified in-process dosage unit sampling and assessment. https://pqri.org/wp-content/uploads/2015/12/FDADraftGuide.pdf
8. Shabushnig, J., & Katayama, H. (2015). Japanese Pharmacopeia (JP) and United States Pharmacopeia (USP) developments in visual inspection for foreign particulate matter. PDA Journal of GMP and Validation in Japan. Retrieved from https://www.jstage.jst.go.jp/article/pda/17/1/17_94/_pdf/-char/ja
9. United States Pharmacopeia (USP). (2020). USP <790>: Visual Inspection of Injections. USP Convention.
10. Savjani, K., Anuradha, G., & Savjani, J. (2012). Drug solubility: importance and enhancement techniques. ISRN Pharmaceutics, 2012, 1-10. https://doi.org/10.5402/2012/195727

11. Lucero-Borja, D., Subirats, X., Barbas, R., Prohens, R., Avdeef, A., & Ràfols, C. (2020). Potentiometric cheqsol and standardized shake-flask solubility methods are complimentary tools in physicochemical profiling. European Journal of Pharmaceutical Sciences, 148, 105305. https://doi.org/10.1016/j.ejps.2020.105305
12. Patil, S. P., Satish, D. V., Peranandhanathan, M., & Mazumdar, D. (2010). Mixing models for slag covered, argon stirred ladles. ISIJ International, 50(8), 1117-1124. https://doi.org/10.2355/isijinternational.50.1117
13. Alam, M. M., E-Zahan, M. K., Rahman, M. H., & Zahid, A. (2020). Water quality assessment of shitalakhya river. Asian Journal of Fisheries and Aquatic Research, 9-20. https://doi.org/10.9734/ajfar/2020/v6i130086
14. Pauline, T., Bouchoud, L., & Bonnabry, P. (2017). Validation of a procedure to mix homogenous solutions in bags and syringes. European Journal of Hospital Pharmacy, 25(e2), e126-e129. https://doi.org/10.1136/ejhpharm-2017-001284
15. Reithmayer, K. (2023, May 2). Accuracy of pH measurement. Xylem. https://www.xylemanalytics.com/en/company/blog/blog/2023/05/accuracy-of-ph-measurement
16. Hamilton. (n.d.). pH accuracy. Hamilton Company. https://www.hamiltoncompany.com/process-analytics/ph-and-orp-knowledge/ph-calibration/ph-accuracy#:~:text=Realistic%20accuracies%20of%20between%20%2B%2F%2D,at%20least%201012%20ohms
17. Fagehi, R., Al-Bishry, A. B., Alanazi, M. A., Abusharha, A., El-Hiti, G. A., & Masmali, A. M. (2021). Investigation of the repeatability of tear osmolarity using an i-pen osmolarity device. Taiwan Journal of Ophthalmology, 11(2), 168. https://doi.org/10.4103/tjo.tjo_65_20
18. Tavakoli, A., Markoulli, M., Flanagan, J., & Papas, E. (2021). The validity of point-of-care tear film osmometers in the diagnosis of dry eye. Ophthalmic and Physiological Optics, 42(1), 140-148. https://doi.org/10.1111/opo.12901
19. U.S. Food and Drug Administration. (2004). Guidance for industry: Sterile drug products produced by aseptic processing – Current good manufacturing practice. U.S. Department of Health and Human Services. https://www.fda.gov/media/71026/download

20. European Medicines Agency. (2014). Guideline on the sterilisation of the medicinal product, active substance, excipient and primary container. EMA/CHMP/CVMP/QWP/BWP/850374/2015. https://www.ema.europa.eu/en/documents/scientific-guideline/guideline-sterilisation-medicinal-product-active-substance-excipient-primary-container_en.pdf
21. Fulton, B., & Gorsky, I. (2024, March/April). Risk- and science-based media and buffer mixing validations. Pharmaceutical Engineering. https://ispe.org/pharmaceutical-engineering/march-april-2024/risk-and-science-based-media-and-buffer-mixing
22. Doran, P. M. (2013). Bioprocess engineering principles (2nd ed.). Academic Press.
23. Benz, G. T. (2021). Agitator design for gas-liquid fermenters and bioreactors (1st ed.). Wiley.
24. Kamps, Á. P., Jödecke, M., Vogt, M., Xia, J., & Maurer, G. (2006). Influence of salts on the solubility of carbon dioxide in (water + methanol). part 2: sodium sulfate. Industrial &Amp; Engineering Chemistry Research, 45(10), 3673-3677. https://doi.org/10.1021/ie0513088
25. Papanyan, Z. K., Roth, C., Wittler, K., Reimann, S., & Ludwig, R. (2013). The dissolution of polyols in salt solutions and ionic liquids at molecular level: ions, counter ions, and Hofmeister effects. ChemPhysChem, 14(16), 3667-3671. https://doi.org/10.1002/cphc.201300465
26. Brauer, A. M., Shi, H., Levin, P. A., & Huang, K. C. (2023). Physiological and regulatory convergence between osmotic and nutrient stress responses in microbes. Current Opinion in Cell Biology, 81, 102170. https://doi.org/10.1016/j.ceb.2023.102170
27. Lu, J. X., Tupper, C., Gutierrez, A. V., & Murray, J. (2022). Biochemistry, Dissolution and Solubility. In StatPearls. StatPearls Publishing.
28. Li, P., Ye, G., Xu, Y., Li, S., Song, L., Li, S., … & Zhou, Q. (2015). Osmolarity affects matrix synthesis in the nucleus pulposus associated with the involvement of mapk pathways: a study of ex vivo disc organ culture system. Journal of Orthopaedic Research, 34(6), 1092-1100. https://doi.org/10.1002/jor.23106

29. Sukhotnik, I., Srugo, I., Lurie, M., Coran, A. G., & Shaoul, R. (2008). Effect of lactulose on bacterial translocation and intestinal adaptation in a rat model of short bowel syndrome. Journal of Pediatric Gastroenterology and Nutrition, 46(5), 507-513. https://doi.org/10.1097/mpg.0b013e31815faa88
30. United States Pharmacopeial Convention. (2012, May 1). USP ⟨811⟩ Powder fineness. United States Pharmacopeia. https://www.usp.org/harmonization-standards/pdg/general-chapters/powder-fineness

Chapter 3: Risk-Based Approach to Determine number of PPQ Runs for Parametric and Non-Parametric attributes

1.0 Introduction

According to the 2011 Process Validation (PV) Guidance Document from the Food and Drug Administration (FDA), "the number of samples [used for PPV] should be adequate to provide sufficient statistical confidence of quality both within a batch and between batches. The confidence level selected can be based on risk analysis as it relates to the particular attribute under examination." [1].

In line with the FDA's guidelines, this article explores two statistical methods for determining the appropriate number of Process Performance Qualification (PPQ) runs for continuous numeric attributes: the Tolerance Interval (TI) method and the Process Capability (PpK) method. For situations involving non-numeric pass/fail results, we discuss the Non-Parametric Binomial and Exponential Chi-Squared methods. Each of these methods offers a way to achieve PPQ results with acceptable statistical confidence, though each comes with its own limitations [2]. Additionally, this article provides detailed, step-by-step instructions for implementing each method using MS Excel.

2.0 Initial Risk Assessment to Determine The Required Level Of Statistical Confidence.

Before calculating the number of PPQ runs, organizations must first assess the risk associated with the attribute or parameter being monitored. The American Society for Testing and Materials (ASTM) outlines three criteria that are used to create a risk assessment matrix for the attributes/parameters to be monitored in PPQ runs: the **severity of the consequences** if a problem or failure occurs, the **likelihood of occurrence**, and the **likelihood of detection** (of a problem or a detection failure).[3] Each of these criteria can then be scored on a scale from 1 to 5, as shown in **Table 1**.

Table 1. Risk assessment scoring matrix based on ASTM recommendations.

Severity (S)	Occurrence (O)	Detectability (D)	Score
Critical process parameter: Directly/indirectly impacts the quality attributes of the product with predefined proven acceptable ranges. Critical quality attributes: Used as the release criteria for the product with predefined specification values.	Most likely to occur	Poor chance of detecting failure	5
Key process parameter (KPP): Parameters that impact the productivity or batch yield with predefined normal operating ranges. In-process controls: Parameters that are monitored at any intermediate stage of the manufacturing process before continuing to the next step with predefined acceptable limits.	Could occur	May detect failure	3
Non-KPP: Typically well-controlled and unlikely to impact the quality or productivity.	Not likely to occur	Will detect failure every time	1

The product of the three scores ((S) x (O) x (D)) gives a "risk priority number (RPN)." Based on the RPN of a given attribute/parameter, the risk associated with that attribute/parameter is classified as high, medium, or low, as shown in Table 2. For each risk classification, Table 2 also shows the International Society for Pharmaceutical Engineering (ISPE) recommendations for setting statistical confidence (1-α) and residual risk (1-p) by defining the proportion of population to cover (p).[14]

Table 2. Guidance for Selecting Statistical Confidence And Population Proportion.

RPN score	Risk classification	Confidence (1-α)/proportion to cover (p) determined by ISPE method
1–25	Low	0.90/0.50
26–50	Medium	0.95/0.70
≥51	High	0.97/0.80

3. Reliability Of the Sample Size Used To Gain Process Knowledge.

The first step in calculating the number of PPQ runs is ensuring the reliability of the sample size used to gain process knowledge. To do this, we can assess the power of estimation as a function of the sample size and a predefined acceptable level of statistical confidence. Equations 1 and 2 show the power of estimation as a function of sample size and confidence for two- and one-sided intervals, respectively:

$$Power\ (1-\beta) = t.dist\left(\left(\frac{\left(\frac{\Delta}{\sigma}\right)}{\sqrt{\frac{1}{n_s}}} - t_{(1-{\alpha}/{2},\ df)}\right), (df)\right) \qquad \text{Eq. (1)}$$

$$Power\ (1-\beta) = t.dist\left(\left(\frac{\left(\frac{\Delta}{\sigma}\right)}{\sqrt{\frac{1}{n_s}}} - t_{(1-\alpha,\ df)}\right), (df)\right) \qquad \text{Eq. (2)}$$

Where t.dist is the cumulative distribution function of the t distribution, n_s is the sample size; df is the degrees of freedom (equal to n_s-1), α is the acceptable type I error rate, β is the acceptable type II error rate, Δ/σ is the detectability or effect size, and $t_{(1-\alpha,\ df)}$ represents the inverse of the cumulative t distribution at 1-α and df.

Here, the significance (α) value or type I error is often set at 0.05,[4] indicating a 5% chance that the null hypothesis is incorrectly rejected (a "false positive"). Detectability (Δ/σ) is expressed as the number of standard deviations that a sample is from the mean. According to the FDA, a detectability of 1.5 at 90% confidence (1-α) is adequate to conclude equivalence between the two groups.[15]

For a confidence level (1-α) of 95%, the widely acceptable minimum power (1-β) is 0.80, [4,16] indicating a 20% chance that the null hypothesis is incorrectly accepted (a "false negative").

4. Tolerance Interval (TI) Method

4.1 Calculating the maximum acceptable tolerance interval

The TI is the range that gives a fixed proportion (p) of the population at a stated statistical confidence (1-α) based on the assumption that the sample data are taken from a normally distributed population.[5, 11] When using the TI method to calculate the required number of PPQ runs, a key parameter is the tolerance interval estimator *k*, which is the number of standard deviations away from the mean that covers a certain fixed proportion of the population at the desired statistical confidence. Accordingly, the maximum acceptable tolerance estimator $k_{max,\ accep}$ is the maximum acceptable *k* value for an acceptable specification, expressed as the maximum acceptable number of standard deviations away from the mean.[12]

One-sided TI. For attributes with one-sided acceptable limits or specification limits, $k_{max,\ accep}$ can be expressed as follows:

$$k_{\max accep} = \frac{SL \pm x_{avg}}{s}$$

Where SL is the specification limit, and X_{avg} and s represent the sample mean and standard deviation, respectively.

Two-sided TI. For attributes with two-sided acceptable limits or specification limits (i.e., an acceptable minimum and an acceptable maximum), the equation for $k_{max,\ accep}$ can be expanded to:

$$k_{\max accep} = maximum\left\{\frac{USL - X_{avg}}{s}, \frac{X_{avg} - LSL}{s}\right\} \qquad \text{Eq. (4)}$$

Where USL is the upper specification limit, and LSL is the lower specification limit.

Accounting for Sample Uncertainty

Because of the limited sample size available before process qualification, we compensate for the uncertainty associated with the sample mean and standard deviation by replacing these values with their respective confidence intervals. The confidence intervals around the mean and standard deviation are shown in Equations 5 and 6.[5]

$$x_{UCI} = x_{avg} + t_{\left(1-\frac{\alpha}{2}, n_s-1\right)} \frac{s}{\sqrt{n_s}}, x_{LCI} = x_{avg} - t_{\left(1-\frac{\alpha}{2}, n_s-1\right)} \frac{s}{\sqrt{n_s}} \qquad \text{Eq. (5)}$$

$$s_{UCI} = s.\sqrt{\frac{n_s - 1}{\chi^2_{(n_s-1),(\alpha)}}} \quad \text{Eq. (6)}$$

Here, x_{UCI} and x_{LCI} represent the upper and lower confidence interval values for the mean, and S_{UCL} represents the upper confidence interval value for the standard deviation.

Substituting Equations 5 and 6 in Equation 4 yields the maximum acceptable tolerance estimator $k_{max,\ accep}$ adjusted for the uncertainty associated with a small sample size:

$$k_{\max accep} = maximum \left\{ \frac{USL - \left(x_{avg} + t_{\left(1-\frac{\alpha}{2}, n_s-1\right)} \frac{s}{\sqrt{n_s}}\right)}{s.\sqrt{\frac{n_s - 1}{\chi^2_{(n_s-1),(\alpha)}}}}, \frac{\left(x_{avg} - t_{\left(1-\frac{\alpha}{2}, n_s-1\right)} \frac{s}{\sqrt{n_s}}\right) -}{s.\sqrt{\frac{n_s - 1}{\chi^2_{(n_s-1),(\alpha)}}}} \right. \quad \text{Eq. (7)}$$

Calculating the tolerance interval for a given specification

One-sided TI. With respect to the true *k* value for a sample, Natreilla (2012) gave an approximate value for *k* for a one-sided TI:[5]

$$k1 = \frac{z_p + \sqrt{z_p^2 - a.b}}{a} \quad \text{Eq. (8)}$$

where

$$a = 1 - \frac{z_\alpha^2}{2(n-1)} \quad \text{Eq. (9)}$$

and

$$b = z_p^2 - \frac{z_\alpha^2}{n} \quad \text{Eq. (10)}$$

Two-sided TI. For a two-sided TI, Howe (1969) expressed the TI estimator k value as a function of sample size (n), confidence (1-α), and proportion (p), as shown in Equation 11.[5]

$$k = z_{\left(\frac{p+1}{2}\right)} \sqrt{\frac{(n-1)(1+\frac{1}{n})}{\chi^2_{\alpha,n-1}}} \qquad \text{Eq. (11)}$$

Where z and χ^2 are the inverse of the cumulative normal distribution and chi-square distribution, respectively.

Later, Guenther corrected Howe's approximation by using k' instead of k for smaller samples, as shown in Equation 12.[5]

$$k' = z_{\left(\frac{p+1}{2}\right)} \sqrt{\frac{(n-1)(1+\frac{1}{n})}{\chi^2_{\alpha,n-1}}} . \sqrt{1+\frac{n-3-\chi^2_{\alpha,n-1}}{2(n+1)^2}} \qquad \text{Eq. (12)}$$

Solving for The Number Of PPQ Runs

The confidence estimator (k1 for a one-sided TI, k' for a two-sided TI) should be less than the maximum confidence limit estimator ($k_{max,accep}$) to ensure that the process remains within the predefined specification limits. The required number of PPQ runs (n) can thus be calculated by finding the value of n at which k1 or k' is approximately equal to but does not exceed, $k_{max,\ accep}$.[11] This condition is shown for k' in Equation 13:

$$k' = z_{\left(\frac{p+1}{2}\right)} \sqrt{\frac{(n-1)(1+\frac{1}{n})}{\chi^2_{\alpha,n-1}}} . \sqrt{1+\frac{n-3-\chi^2_{\alpha,n-1}}{2(n+1)^2}} \leq k_{\max accep}$$

Eq. (13)

Process Capability Method

Defining the process performance index (P_{pK})

The ability of a process to meet predefined specifications is determined by the process performance index (P_{pK}), which is defined as the ratio of the distance from the process mean and nearest specification to the one-sided spread of the process (3σ variation) based on the overall standard deviation for a normally distributed population.[6] P_{pK} is calculated as shown in Equation 14:[7]

$$P_{pK} = minimum\{PpU\,, PpL\}$$

$$= minimum\left\{\frac{USL-\mu}{3\sigma}, \frac{\mu - LSL}{3\sigma}\right\} \qquad \text{Eq. (14)}$$

Where P_{pK} is the process performance index, PpL is the lower process performance index, and PpU is the upper process performance index. PpL and PpU can be expressed in terms of the upper and lower specification limits, as shown in Equation 14. μ and σ represent the underlying true population mean and the overall true population standard deviation, respectively.

Accounting for sample uncertainty

The above equation for P_{pK} (Eq. 14) is typically employed when the sample size is at least 25. However, the sample size generated before the process qualification phase is often less than 25, creating a degree of uncertainty around the underlying true population mean and standard deviation. As discussed for the TI method, this uncertainty can be compensated for by replacing the sample mean and sample standard deviation with their respective confidence intervals.

The sigma factor of ±3 in the 3σ term in Equation 14 represents the number of standard deviations from the mean that covers 99.7% of the true population. However, (i) the proportion of the population to cover is determined based on the risk assessment, and (ii) we must account for the uncertainty involved in a limited available sample size. For these reasons, the term ±3 in Equation 14 is replaced with the variable *r* in Equation 17. *r* represents the number of sigma factors from the mean that cover the desired proportion of the population.

By substituting Equations 5 and 6 into Equation 14 and replacing ±3 with *r*, the equation for P_{pK} can be rewritten as follows:

$$P_{pK} = min\left\{\frac{USL - \left(x_{avg} + t_{\left(1-\frac{\alpha}{2}, n_s-1\right)}\frac{s}{\sqrt{n_s}}\right)}{r.s.\sqrt{\frac{n_s-1}{\chi^2_{(n_s-1),(\alpha)}}}}, \frac{\left(x_{avg} - t_{\left(1-\frac{\alpha}{2}, n_s-1\right)}\frac{s}{\sqrt{n_s}}\right) - LSL}{r.s.\sqrt{\frac{n_s-1}{\chi^2_{(n_s-1),(\alpha)}}}}\right\} \quad \text{Eq. (15)}$$

The r value can be calculated iteratively by increasing the value of k from k=0 in Equation 10 to achieve the desired population proportion based on the risk assessment.

$$p = \left(NORM.S.DIST\left(\frac{1}{\sqrt{n_s}} + r\right), TRUE\right) - \left(NORM.S.DIST\left(\frac{1}{\sqrt{n_s}} - r\right), TRUE\right) \quad \text{Eq. (16)}$$

Equation 17 gives Bissell's approximation of the confidence interval for a capability index (PpK) that accounts for the uncertainty in the sample:[8, 9, 10]

$$P_{pK} - Z_{1-\alpha}\sqrt{\frac{1}{k^2 n} + \frac{P_{pK}^2}{2(n-1)}} \leq Ppk \leq P_{pK} - Z_{1-\alpha}\sqrt{\frac{1}{k^2 n} + \frac{P_{pK}^2}{2(n-1)}} \quad \text{Eq. (17)}$$

Solving for the number of PPQ runs.

According to the FDA's 2011 PV guidance, a capability index value of 1.0–1.3 indicates that a process is capable and most likely to meet the specifications routinely.[7] We, therefore, need to determine the number of PPQ runs required for the lower bound of P_{pK}, also known as the lower capability confidence interval (LCCI), to be approximately 1.0–1.3.

Sample sizes <30. For smaller sample sizes, the required number of process validation batches (n) can be determined by iteratively increasing the value of n in Equation 18 (starting from 3) until LCCI is 1.0–1.3.

$$LCCI = P_{pK} - Z_{1-\alpha}\sqrt{\frac{1}{k^2 n} + \frac{P_{pK}^2}{2(n-1)}} \geq 1.0 \qquad \text{Eq. (18)}$$

Sample sizes ≥30. When the available sample size is ≥30, we can use Wu and Kuo's (2004) method for calculating the LCCI. In this method, Equation 18 is simplified by replacing k with 3. The equation is then rearranged to directly solve for the number of PPQ runs (*n*) needed to meet the predefined specification at a specified confidence level (α):[9]

$$n = \frac{z_{\alpha}^{2}\left(\left(\frac{1}{9P_{pK}}\right) + 0.5\right)}{\left(1 - \frac{LCCI}{P_{pK}}\right)^2} \qquad \text{Eq. (19)}$$

Non-parametric Method

If the monitored parameter does not follow any specific data distribution or results reports as pass/fail; then the statistical approach for the selection of sample size to ensure the reliability of the effectiveness check is not necessarily straightforward. Therefore, this article also details one such appropriate statistical approach to calculate the sample size named "Reliability Demonstration Tests" (RDT) to verify whether a product/process has met a certain reliability requirement at a stated statistical confidence level when the underlying data distribution is unknown.

Different RTD methods (Cumulative Binomial, Non-Parametric Binomial, Exponential Chi-Squared and Non-Parametric Bayesian) are available. This article focuses on two of the simplest and easy to adopt methods, named Non-Parametric Binomial and Exponential Chi-Squared methods, as the rest of the methods have limitations, such as feeding prior information based on assumptions, and there is no one "correct way of calculating prior information" and different approaches give different results. Furthermore, this article also recommends risk assessment methodology for the selection of acceptable reliability and statistical confidence that may be used in the above discussed two RDT methods.

Non-Parametric Binomial Method:

This method is also called the Classical Reliability Demonstration Test. When "x" is the number of observed failures out of "n" trials. And the probability of each trial "p" is an independent Bernoulli trial. Then, the probability of at least "c" failure can be calculated using binomial distribution [17].

$$Prob\ \{obataining\ \text{"c" or}\ less\ failures\} = \sum_{x=0}^{c} C_x^n \times p^x (1-p)^{n-x} \quad \text{Eq. (20)}$$

For zero failures, assuming "c" = 0, the above equation-20 reduces to equation 21:

$$Prob\ \{zero\ occorence, \text{"}c = 0\text{"}\} = (1-p)^n \quad \text{Eq. (21)}$$

(1-p) is also termed as reliability (R).

Equation 21 can be re-written as:

$$(1-p)^n = R^n \qquad \text{Eq. (22)}$$

Now, the number sample size can be determined by equating equation-22 to significance value (α) type-1 error, in other words probability of falsely rejecting a true null hypothesis.

$$(1-p)^n = R^n \geq \alpha \qquad \text{Eq. (23)}$$

Taking Logarithms on both sides in the above equation 4 and solving for sample size (n), we obtain:

$$n \geq \frac{ln(\alpha)}{ln(R)} = \frac{ln(1-C)}{ln\ (R)} \qquad \text{Eq. (24)}$$

In the above equation 24, the term "C" is confidence. Equation 5 tells us to have C % confidence, and the CAPA is R % reliable. A minimum of n samples needs to be tested to ensure zero failure as acceptance criteria.

Exponential Chi-Squared Method:

In an exponential chi-squared method, the sample size for zero failure is again calculated as a function of reliability and confidence, as shown in equation 25 [17].

$$n \geq \frac{\chi^2_{(1-C,2)}}{2 \times (1-R)} \qquad \text{Eq. (25)}$$

Where,

χ2(1-C, 2) represents the inverse of the right-tailed probability of the chi-squared distribution at 1-C probability and "2" degrees of freedom. In Microsoft Excel, this value can be calculated using =CHISQ.INV.RT (probability, degrees of freedom) function.

Risk Assessment: The risk associated with the attribute/parameter is classified as high, medium, or low, as shown in Table 2. For each risk classification, Table 2 also shows the recommendations for Confidence (C) and Reliability. The selection of reliability is based on Rules of thumb on Cronbach`s Alpha coefficient that measures the measures' reliability, or internal consistency [17].

Table 3. Guidance for selecting statistical confidence and population proportion.

RPN score	Risk classification	Confidence (1-C)	Reliability (R)	Number of samples required based on the Non-Parametric Binomial Method	Number of samples required based on the Exponential Chi-Squared Method
1–25	Low	0.90	0.60*	5	6
26–50	Medium	0.90	0.70 *	6	8
≥ 51	High	0.95	0.80	13	15
0.6 And 0.7 reliability scores are acceptable based on the assumption that the control strategy for failure mode is well reliable and only the statistical confidence in the corrective action implemented needs to be demonstrated.					

Conclusion

Understanding both the process and the product is achieved through data from the initial phases of process development, past experiences with similar processes, scale-up efforts, scale-down model validation runs, and process characterization studies [10]. However, new therapeutic technologies, such as gene-modified ex vivo cell-based therapies and in vitro gene therapies, introduce unique challenges to the process validation workflow. Whereas traditional approaches relied on three production batches for process qualification in the case of biologics and small molecules, these emerging therapies require a risk-based methodology to determine the number of Process Performance Qualification (PPQ) runs needed to meet predefined specifications with a certain level of statistical confidence.

For determining sample sizes in cases where pass/fail results are non-numeric, both the Non-Parametric Binomial and Exponential Chi-Squared methods are widely accepted practices in FDA-regulated industries. As demonstrated in Table 3, there is no significant difference between the sample sizes calculated using these two approaches, so either method can be used.

The concepts of confidence and reliability discussed in this article are meant for illustrative purposes. However, depending on the specifics of the process, batch production rate, and associated costs, it is strongly recommended that drug manufacturers select confidence and reliability values that are more appropriate for their quality policies and practices.

References

1. U.S. Department of Health and Human Services Food and Drug Administration. (2011, January). Guidance for Industry Process Validation: General Principles and Practices. http://www.fda.gov/downloads/Drugs/Guidances/UCM070336.pdf

2. James, D., Nesta, D. P., Desai, K. D., & Lewis, R. A. (2017, June 30). Stage 2 Process Validation: Regulatory Expectations and Approaches to Determine and Justify the Number of PPQ Batches. Biopharma International, 30(7).

3. ASTM E2476-09 Standard Guide for Risk Assessment and Risk Control as it Impacts the Design, Development, and Operation of PAT Processes for Pharmaceutical Manufacture.

4. Lakens, D. (2013). Calculating and reporting effect sizes to facilitate cumulative science: A practical primer for T-TesTs and ANOVAs. Frontiers in Psychology, 4. https://doi.org/10.3389/fpsyg.2013.00863

5. NIST/SEMATECH. (2012). Handbook of Statistical Methods. NIST. https://doi.org/10.18434/M32189

6. Cohen, J. (1988). Statistical Power Analysis for the Behavioral Sciences (2nd ed.). LAWRENCE ERLBAUM ASSOCIATES.

7. *Utilization of statistical methods for production monitoring*. (2012). Parenteral Drug Association. https://www.pda.org/bookstore/product-detail/1842-tr-59-utilization-of-statistical-methods

8. Charoo, N. A. (2018). Estimating number of PPQ batches: Various approaches. Journal of Pharmaceutical Innovation, 13(2), 188-196. https://doi.org/10.1007/s12247-018-9316-2

9. Wu, C. C., & Kuo, H. L. (2004). Sample Size Determination for the Estimate of Process Capability Indices. Information and Management Sciences, 15(1), 1-12.

10. Yang, H. (2016). Emerging non-clinical biostatistics in Biopharmaceutical development and manufacturing. CRC Press.

11. Durivage, M. (2016, October 27). How To Establish Sample Sizes For Process Validation Using Statistical Tolerance Intervals. Bioprocess Online.

12. Vasta, A. (2021). Determining sample size for specification limits verification with tolerance intervals. Quality and Reliability Engineering International, 37(5), 1718-1739. https://doi.org/10.1002/qre.2821

13. Bryder, M., Etling, H., Fleming, J., Hu, Y., & Levy, P. (2014, February 1). Topic 1 – Stage 2 Process Validation: Determining and Justifying the Number of Process Performance Qualification Batches (version 2). ISPE | International Society for Pharmaceutical Engineering. https://ispe.org/publications/papers/stage-2-process-validation-process-performance-qualification-batches

14. Weng, Y. (2016). STATISTICAL REVIEW AND EVALUATION (Reference ID: 4026576). FDA. https://www.fda.gov/media/105013/download

15. Schuirmann, D. J. (1987). A comparison of the two one-sided test procedures and the power approach for assessing the equivalence of average bioavailability. Journal of Pharmacokinetics and Biopharmaceutics, 15(6), 657-680. https://doi.org/10.1007/bf01068419

16. Heidaran M. (2019, April 25). Manufacturing Controls at Commercial Scale: A Major Hurdle for the Cell and Gene Therapy Industry. Regulatory Focus. https://www.raps.org/news-and-articles/news-articles/2019/4/establishing-manufacturing-controls-a-hurdle-for

17. Muralidharan, N. (1), Lorson, D., (2024, January/February). Determining Sample Size for Demonstrating Zero Failures Ensuring the Effectiveness of Corrective and Preventive Actions. Bioprocess International, 22(1-2). https://bioprocessintl.com/analytical/qa-qc/determiningsample-size-for-demonstrating-zero-failures-ensuring-the-effectiveness-of-corrective-andpreventive-actions/

Chapter 4: Understanding Sources of Variability in Analytical Methods and the Use of Statistical Interval Methods to Define Different Acceptable Limits

1. Introduction

Maintaining compliance with the regulations of institutions such as the U.S. Food and Drug Administration (FDA) and the European Medicines Agency (EMA) is critical for rationally regulated pharmaceutical and biopharmaceutical drug manufacture. In biopharmaceuticals, the most commonly used terminologies describing situations where data fall outside of historic expectations are out-of-statistical control (OOSC), out-of-trend (OOT), out-of-specification (OOS), and out-of-expectation (OOE). FDA Form 483, published on 26th April 2023, stated that inadequate investigation was performed on OOS and OOT results, with companies routinely invalidating them by re-testing batches without a scientifically justified reason for invalidating the original result [1].

Invalidating a reported analytical test result requires a sound understanding of assay and process variability. Therefore, in the present article, we detail how the accuracy and precision of analytical methods are assessed, and we discuss what statistical methods are appropriate means by which to establish the validity of an analytical run. Furthermore, while OOS results indicate a failure to meet predefined limits, ambiguity remains with the definitions of OOE, OOSC, and OOT and how they differ, largely due to a lack of systematic study [2]. Accordingly, in the present article, we delineate OOE, OOSC, and OOT, how they differ, and what appropriate statistical approaches are used to establish these limits.

2. Different limit terminologies used in biopharmaceuticals

2.1 OOS

OOS refers to a situation where a product, component, or material does not meet predetermined specifications or acceptance criteria. It indicates a deviation from established quality standards, such as that in terms of potency, purity, identity, or other relevant parameter [3].

2.2 OOE and OOSC

Both these terms concern variability in reported results, but in different ways. Any reported product-analysis result is susceptible to variability, often referred to as overall observed variability (σ_O^2), which has contributions from manufacturing-process variability (σ_m^2) and variability in the assay method itself (σ_a^2), as detailed in Eq. (1) [4].

$$\sigma_O{}^2 = \sigma_m{}^2 + \sigma_A{}^2 \tag{1}$$

A result that meets specifications but is outside the expected overall observed variability (σ_O^2) is defined as OOT/OOSC. A result that meets specifications but is outside the expected variability of the analytical method (σ_a^2) is defined as OOE. Both OOT and OOSC results serve as early warning signs of potential compliance risks violating specification limits. Identifying deviations from expected historical performance helps manufacturers to proactively investigate their products if necessary and address any underlying issues before they escalate into major specification violations. Conversely, OOE serves as an acceptance criterion for an analytical run [5]. The results of an analytical test for a specific batch may or may not meet release specifications. However, they may also fail to meet the acceptable variability of the analytical test method. In such instances, the analytical test cannot be used to support either the acceptance or rejection of the batch. OOE results warrant reinvestigation and sample reanalysis.

3. Analytical method performance characteristics to monitor variability

USP standard <1225> states that if measurements are susceptible to variations in analytical conditions, these should be suitably controlled in the procedure [6]. The International Council for Harmonization of Technical Requirements (ICH) guideline M10 on bioanalytical method validation states that criteria for the acceptance or rejection of an analytical test run should be defined. The acceptability criteria of an assay should be based on statistically derived variability in historic data. The variability of analytical test methods is monitored in two different ways: by running replicates of the same sample and by running known standards along with a sample [7].

3.1 Running replicates of samples

In this methodology, a single sample or standard is measured more than once, so any measured variable is inherent to the variability of the analytical method itself. Therefore, USP <1010> advocates for the use of statistical methods to judge the true value of any measured variable [8]. Hence, in biopharmaceuticals, samples are often analyzed in replications, and the averages of discrete measurements are reported to give more reliable results. Per USP <1010>, the degree of agreement among individual test results when the analytical method is applied repeatedly to a homogeneous sample is termed 'precision' [8]. The acceptable variability limits within the replicates are statistically derived during method development. Agreement between replicates is expressed as a percentage relative standard deviation (%RSD). If (x) is the random variable, and ($\bar{x}$) and (S) are the sample average value and sample standard deviation, respectively, from samples $X_{i=1}$, $X_{i=2}$, $X_{i=3}$...$X_{i=n}$ with a sample size of n, then %RSD is calculated using Eqs. (2) to (4). Tiwari et al. (2010) reported that for typical assay methods, the RSD must be ≤ 2.0%, while the acceptance criteria for impurities are dependent on the level of impurity and the sensitivity of the method [9].

$$\%RSD = \frac{S}{\bar{x}}.100 \tag{2}$$

Where,

$$\bar{x} = \frac{\sum_{i=i}^{i=n} x_i}{n} \tag{3}$$

and

$$\boldsymbol{S} = \sqrt{\sum_{i=i}^{i=n} \frac{(x_i - \bar{x})^2}{n-1}} \tag{4}$$

The most common approach to setting the acceptance criteria between replicates for the same sample, or precision, can be calculated as the upper confidence bound (UCB) on sample standard deviation, as shown in (5).

$$UCB_S = \sqrt{\frac{(n-1).S}{\chi^2_{\propto,n-1}}} \qquad (5)$$

ICH Q2 (R1) Validation of Analytical Procedures further subdivides precision into three levels [10].

- **Repeatability**: Expresses the precision under the same operating conditions over a short interval of time. Repeatability is also termed intra-assay precision. Repeatability should be assessed for early-phase method qualification. ICH documents recommend repeatability be assessed using a minimum of nine determinations covering a specified range or using a minimum of six determinations at 100% concentration of the analyte [11].

- **Intermediate precision:** Expresses within-laboratories variations: different days, different analysts, and different equipment, which is typically performed during late Phase 2 or Phase 3 of a drug's development [12].

- **Reproducibility:** Expresses the precision between laboratories (collaborative studies, usually applied to standardization of methodology). Applicable when multiple sites are used for analytical testing.

3.2 Running known standards

Often, replicates of known standards are used in assays to ensure their accuracy and precision are within predefined validated ranges. Either single standard concentration or multi-level standards (where the original weighing standard is diluted to prepare a series of standards over a range of concentrations) are used.

Type of Assay	QC standard Requirement ICH M10
Ligand Binding Assay	An analytical run consists of a blank sample, at least 6 calibration standard concentration levels, at least 3 QCs in duplicate (or 5% of the number of samples) and the study samples.
Chromatography Assay	An analytical run consists of a blank sample, a zero sample, at least 6 calibration standard concentration levels, at least 3 QCs in duplicate (or 5% of the number of samples) and the study samples

USP <1225> states that the accuracy of an analytical procedure is the closeness of test results obtained by that procedure to the known true value [6]. In biopharmaceuticals, samples are analyzed in replicate, which forms a distribution of data, and the true value is estimated from the average of the replicates. However, simply measuring the deviation between a known standard and the mean estimate of replicates does not consider the uncertainty from variability within replicates (precision).

The International Standard Organization (ISO) definition of accuracy is different from that in USP <1225>. For the ISO, the term accuracy combines deviation from the known true value and precision together. Therefore, the region of uncertainty or offset in the measured assay result is often measured as a combination of both accuracy and recession [11]. Furthermore, when a known single standard is used in the assay, the term "recovery" is used to assess the variability between actual known concentrations. When a multi-level standard is used, linearity is used to evaluate the variability of the assay method [12]. USP <1225> states that the linearity of an analytical procedure refers to the relationship between an actual known concentration to a measured concentration. If a linear model is not attainable, a non-linear model can be acceptable. Here, the closeness in the relationship between the predicted and actual values is most important. Furthermore, USP <1225> also states that any analytical method with a defined measurement range should be demonstrated to have acceptable levels of precision, accuracy, and recovery/linearity. Figure 1 demonstrates the relationship between accuracy and precision [6].

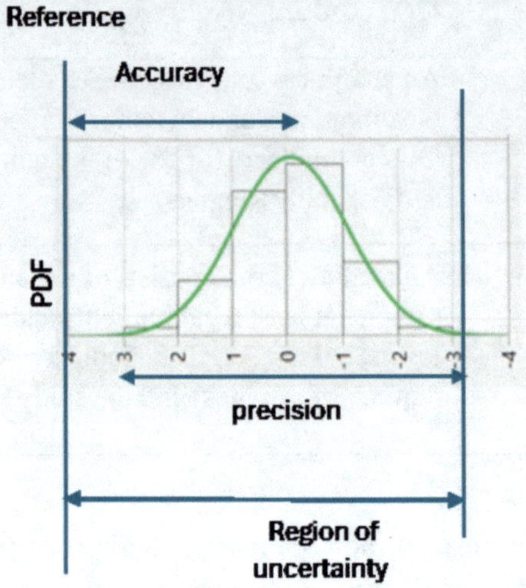

3.3 Defining Acceptance Criteria.

3.3.1 Accuracy and precision

Tolerance intervals have been recommended for simultaneously validating both the accuracy and precision of an analytical procedure, as shown in Eqs. (6) and (7) [11, 12].

$$TI = [\bar{x} \pm k.S] \tag{6}$$

$$k = \sqrt{\frac{z^2_{\frac{1+p}{2}} \cdot (n-1)}{\chi^2_{\alpha,n-1}}\left(1+\frac{1}{n}\right)} \tag{7}$$

Acceptance criteria for accuracy and precision based on the type of analytical method recommended by ICH M(10) afre summarized in Table 1 [13].

Table 1. Acceptance criteria for accuracy and precision

Type of Assay	Acceptance Criteria for Accuracy and Precision
Ligand Binding Assay	The calibration standard should be within ±25% of the nominal concentration at the LLOQ and ULOQ and ±20% at all other levels.
Chromatography Assay	The back-calculated concentrations of the calibration standards should be within ±15% of the nominal value, except for the LLOQ, for which it should be within ±20%. At least 75% of the calibration standard concentrations, which should include a minimum of six concentration levels, should fulfill these criteria.

3.3.2 Ruggedness factor

The concept of using an upper confidence interval on standard deviation (as shown in Eq. (5)) to assess precision is only applicable at the repeatability level [11]. However, for intermediate precision and reproducibility, precision incorporates 'ruggedness factor' as shown in Eq. (8). Here, S_{IP}^2 is variability in intermediate precession, and S_R^2 is variability from repeatability (i.e., variability in assay results when conducted under the same conditions), and S_{RD}^2 is ruggedness variability, also referred as ruggedness factor (i.e., this is the variability from changes in reagent batch and analyst).

$$S_{IP}{}^2 = S_R{}^2 + S_{RD}{}^2 \quad (8)$$

	Analyst			
Result	A1	A2	A3	A4
R1	X_{R1A1}	X_{R1A2}	X_{R1A3}	X_{R1A4}
R2	X_{R2A1}	X_{R2A2}	X_{R2A3}	X_{R2A4}
R3	X_{R3A1}	X_{R3A2}	X_{R3A3}	X_{R3A4}
Average	Avg_{A1}	Avg_{A2}	Avg_{A3}	Avg_{A4}
Std Dev	S_{A1}	S_{A2}	S_{A3}	S_{A4}

Variance from repeatability is assessed as expressed in Eq. (9).

$$S_R^2 = \frac{S_{A1}^2 + S_{A2}^2 + S_{A3}^3 + S_{A4}^3}{4} \quad (9)$$

Estimation variance from ruggedness factor is determined using the approach as summarized in Eq. (10). If we assume "n = 3" is the number of times a sample is analyzed under each analyst, "I = 4" is the number of different analysts used in ruggedness factor assessment, and "N = 12" is the total number of reported results. Now, $\bar{x}_{all}$ is the average of all the reported results (Sum of all 12 results reported divided by N = 12), and $\bar{x}_{Ai}$ is the average for four analysts ([Avg_{A1} + Avg_{A1} + Avg_{A1} + Avg_{A1}] ÷ 4).

$$S_{RD}^2 = \frac{\sum_{i=1}^{i=4}(\bar{x}_{Ai} - \bar{x}_{all})^2}{(i-1)} - \frac{S_R^2}{n} \quad (10)$$

Now, the variability in an assay result combined from accuracy and intermediate precision (in intermediate and precision and precision level repeatability) is given by the modified tolerance interval, as expressed in Eqs(11) to (12).

$$TI = [\bar{x} \pm k_{IP}.S_{IP}] \tag{11}$$

$$k_{IP} = \sqrt{\frac{\left(1 + \frac{1}{i+n}\right) Z^2_{(1+p)/2} \times df}{\chi^2_{(2\alpha),df}}} \tag{12}$$

$$df = \frac{(S_{IP})^4}{\frac{\left[\sum_{i=1}^{i=4}(\bar{x}_{Ai} - \bar{x}_{all})^2\right]^2}{(i-1)^3} + \frac{(n-1) \times S_R^4}{n^2 \times i}} \tag{13}$$

3.3.3 Recovery

When a one-level standard concentration is used to assess the accuracy, recovery (%R) is used to evaluate the relationship between the estimated and actual concentrations, as shown in Eq. (14). Here, X_C is the known standard concentration, and Y_C is the measured concentration. The FDA Regulatory Affairs Laboratory Manual II states that the general acceptance criteria of recovery for human drug analytical methods is 80%–120% [12].

$$(\%R) = \frac{Y_C}{X_C} \tag{14}$$

3.3.4 Linearity

When a multi-level standard is used, the linear correlation model between the predicted concentration (Y_C) and known standard concentration (X_C) takes the form shown in Eq. (15).

$$Y_C = b.X_C + a \tag{15}$$

For a linear fit, the slope (b) and intercept (a) are expected around zero and one, respectively. However, the linear predictive model is still susceptible to some variability. Therefore, the acceptance criteria for a slope in a linear regression model is given by a two-sided confidence interval at a pre-set acceptable risk (α) using Eqs. (16) to (18), as shown by Funk (2007) [14]. Here, the significance (α) value or type I error is often set at an acceptable value of 0.05 [4], indicating a 5% chance of false rejection of an actually true null hypothesis or, in other words, a 5% chance of incorrectly concluding a difference when there is none. Now, statistical confidence is defined as (1 – α), that is, 100% – 5% = 95% [15].

ICH Q2 recommends that, for the establishment of linearity, a minimum of five concentrations should normally be used. It is also recommended that the following minimum specified ranges should be considered: Assay of a drug substance (or a finished product): from 80% to 120% of the test concentration; determination of an impurity: from 50% to 120% of the acceptance criterion; content uniformity: a minimum of 70% to 130% of the test concentration, unless a wider or more appropriate range based on the nature of the dosage form is justified [16].

$$CI_b = b \pm t_{1-\frac{\alpha}{2},n-2} \times \frac{S_y}{\sqrt{Q_{xx}}} \tag{16}$$

Here,

$$S_y = \sqrt{\frac{\sum Y_{c,i} - (a + b.X_{c,i})^2}{n-2}}; Q_{XX} = \sum X_{c,i}{}^2 - \frac{1}{n}\left(\sum X_{c,i}\right)^2 \quad (17)$$

$$CI_a = a \pm t_{1-\frac{\alpha}{2},n-2}.S_y.\sqrt{\frac{1}{n} + \frac{\bar{X}^2}{Q_{XX}}} \quad (18)$$

4.0 OOT and OOSC limits

The FDA's 2011 Process Validation Guidance recommends continued process verification (CPV) during stage-3 process monitoring for drug manufacturers. In CPV, Shewhart control charts are employed as a statistical tool for monitoring process parameters and attributes to identify OOT and OOSC. In control charts, the calculated process average is utilized as the center line, and control limits are placed at a distance k = ±3 short-term standard deviations (σ_R) away from the process average. The control chart, along with Nelson rules, serves as a tool for detecting OOSC data, defined as data that fall beyond the set control limits, and OOT data, defined as a group of data that forms a non-random pattern (shift in mean or increasing/decreasing pattern) [17-19].

4.1 Response to violation of OOT and OOSC limits

OOT and OOSC may not instantaneously warrant an investigation or a corrective action under the quality system employed. However, during a data review, the identified statistical process control signals for OOT or OOSC are disused in terms of 1) magnitude of the signal, 2) statistical reliability of signal, and 3) risk (and severity) to product quality or/and process performance. The decision on how to respond to the signal must be warranted. If the signal is identified as a nascent signal or not practically or statistically significant enough, then no response or action is required. If the signal is identified to be real and has both practical and statistical strength but is still not significant enough to impact product quality, then a technical evaluation may be warranted to understand the cause of variation better. Details of such evaluations and results should be followed up in subsequent CPV meetings, and their findings should be documented in CPV meeting minutes. If the signal is identified to be real, has both practical and statistical significance, and the magnitude is significant enough to impact the product quality potentially, then an investigation under the quality management system may be required [15].

4.2 Control charts

In 1924, Walter Andrew Shewhart introduced the concept of data analysis using control charts, which was later adopted by the pharmaceutical and biopharmaceutical industries when regulatory agencies requested that drug manufacturers perform CPV [20]. In control charts or XBar charts, the center line is placed at the average, and control limits are typically placed at k standard deviations from the average. Typically, $k = 3$ is utilized, for which there is a 0.135% probability that any data point belonging to a normally distributed population will fall outside ± 3 standard deviations (σ). This approach gives an interval of expected future observations if the process does not change. If observations are within these limits, it can be assumed that the validated state is maintained; if observations are outside these limits, the mean and/or standard deviation has probably changed, potentially requiring attention. σ is often calculated as a short-term σR, which causes the limits to be more sensitive to drift, as expressed in Eq. (19).

$$CL = \mu \pm 3(\sigma_R) \tag{19}$$

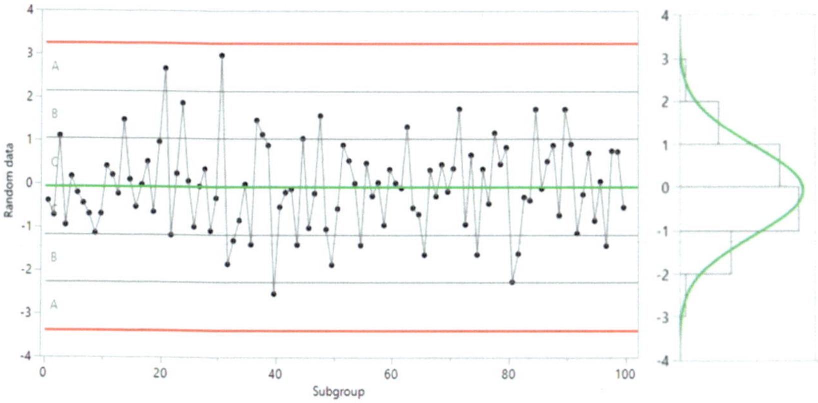

The control chart is divided into six zones based on distance from the center line, as shown in Figure 2. Each zone is one standard deviation (σ_R) wide. The 3-σ_R limits to both sides of the center line show the upper control limit and lower control limit. The 2-σ_R limits indicate the upper and lower warning limits, and the 1-σR limits on each side of the center line are the upper and lower one-sigma limits. Control charts, along with Nelson rules 1–8, are used to monitor process control and process stability based on the location of data in different zones, the frequency of occurrence of any patterns, and the distance from the mean [20]. In statistical process control, the FAR, or rate of type-I errors, often identified by the symbol α, indicates the likelihood that data will be falsely identified as an abnormal signal when the data actually correspond to the normal variability of the process. Table 2 summarizes the different Nelson rules and their purposes, along with the probability of a false alarm for each Nelson rule [20].

Table 2. Nelson's rules and their purposes

Test number	**Purpose**
Rule 1: One data point outside the control limit	Detect OOSC data.
Rule 2: Nine consecutive data points on one side of the center line	Detect a process shift.

Test number	Purpose
Rule 3: Six consecutive data points either increasing or decreasing	Detect a process drift.
Rule 4: Fourteen consecutive data points alternating up and down	Detect a process alternating between two states.
Rule 5: Two out of three data points falling outside two sigmas from the center line	Detect an intermediate shift.
Rule 6: Four out of five data points falling outside two sigmas from the center line	Detect a small shift.
Rule 7: Fifteen data points falling within one sigma from the center line	Detect a reduction in process variability.
Rule 8: Eight consecutive data points falling outside one sigma from the center line	Detect mixed process behavior.

The FARs from all eight Nelson rules identified in Table 2 total 2.65%. Although it might be intriguing to use all eight Nelson test rules, Nelson (1984) suggested keeping the FAR below 1% [20]. Nelson also stated that tests 5 and 6 should be included only when there is an economic desire to have an early warning, as these rules increase the FAR. Tests 7 and 8 are used to diagnose stratifications and to identify subgroups taken from two different means. Therefore, test rules 7 and 8 have application only when subgroups are used in the control chart. However, in the biopharmaceutical industry, testing is typically performed for a single sample taken from a batch; therefore, unless multiple samples are tested and averaged for the single value reported in the control chart, rules 7 and 8 do not add value for data monitoring and trending. Adhibhatta et al. (2017) showed that Nelson tests 1 to 4 are adequate for monitoring OOSC and OOT data, with a combined false alarm probability of 0.94 [21]. Thus, in an effort to limit the FAR to < 1.0% and considering the practical application of test rules for biopharmaceuticals, it is recommended that only Nelson test rules 1–3 be utilized in a control chart for biopharmaceutical application.

5.0 Conclusions

In biopharmaceuticals, process limits such as OOE, OOSC, and OOT are often used. However, their similarities and differences are often misunderstood. Therefore, in this article, we have detailed their resemblances and distinctions. Furthermore, we have also detailed the statistical approaches and tools used to define these limits. Additionally, throughout the article we have cited regulatory expectations along with appropriate usage.

References

1. Foreign Manufacturing Sites Inspection Records. U.S. Food and Drug Administration, 12 Apr. 2024, www.fda.gov/drugs/cder-foia-electronic-reading-room/frequently-requested-or-proactively-posted-compliance-records.

2. Torbeck, L. "OOS, OOT, OOC, and OOSC." PharmTech, 1 Oct. 2011, www.pharmtech.com/view/oos-oot-ooc-and-oosc.

3. Investigating Out-of-Specification (OOS) Test Results for Pharmaceutical Production Guidance for Industry. U.S. Food and Drug Administration. 2022, www.fda.gov/media/158416/download.

4. Ott, Lyman, and Michael Longnecker. An Introduction to Statistical Methods and Data Analysis. Cengage Learning, 2010.

5. Burgess, C. LABORATORY DATA MANAGEMENT GUIDANCE Out of Expectation (OOE) and Out of Trend (OOT) Results. Analytical Quality Control Working Group, 2016. Accessed 15 Apr. 2024. https://www.scribd.com/document/511521881/Laboratory-Data-Management-Guidance

6. USP44-NF39 2021, General Chapters, General Test and Assay, <1225> Validation of Compendial procedure (accessed February 22, 2022), p 1–12, https://online.uspnf.com/uspnf/document/1_GUIDE2C6F9E8-EA71-4B72-A7BA-76ABD5E72964_4_en-US

7. European Medicines Agency ICH guideline M10 2019 on bioanalytical method validation, European Medicines Agency. https://www.ema.europa.eu/en/documents/scientific -guideline/draft-ich-guideline-m10-bioanalyticalmethod-validation-step-2b_en.pdf

8. USP44-NF39 2021, General Chapters, General Test and Assay, <1010> Analytical Data – Interpretation and Treatment), p 1–29. https://online.uspnf.com/uspnf/document/1_GUID5C0818CD-E76F-44B8-B504-C202CA762F2A_5_en-US

9. Tiwari G, Tiwari R. Bioanalytical method validation: An updated review. Pharm Methods. 2010;1(1):25-38. https://www.ncbi.nlm.nih.gov/pmc/articles/PMC3658022/

10. European Medicines Agency ICH Q2 (R2) 2022, Validation of the Analytical Procedure (accessed September 22, 2022), https://www.ema.europa.eu/en/documents/scientific-guideline/ich-guideline-q2r2-validation-analytical-procedures-step-2b_en.pdf

11. Coffey, T., & Yang, H. (2018). Statistics for biotechnology process development. CRC Press.

12. Application of accuracy and precision evaluations based on the current United States and Indonesian pharmacopoeias: A critical review. (2022). Makara Journal of Science, 26(4). https://doi.org/10.7454/mss.v26i4.1343

13. European Medicines Agency ICH guideline M10 2019 on bioanalytical method validation, European Medicines Agency. https://www.ema.europa.eu/en/documents/scientific-guideline/draft-ich-guideline-m10-bioanalyticalmethod-validation-step-2b_en.pdf

14. Funk, W., Dammann, V., Donnevert, G. 2007. Quality Assurance in the Analytical Chemistry, 2nd ed. Wiley–VCH Verlag GmbH & Co. KGaA. Weinheim Germany. pp. 12–43; 236–238.

15. Muralidharan N, Johnson T, Rose LS, Davis M. CPV Monitoring - Optimization of Control Chart Design by Reducing the False Alarm Rate and Nuisance Signal. Sci J Appl Math Stat. 2024;12(2):20-28. https://www.sciencepublishinggroup.com/article/10.11648/j.sjam

16. European Medicines Agency ICH Q2 (R1) 2006, Validation of analytical procedures: text and methodology, (accessed April 22, 2024), https://www.fda.gov/regulatory-information/search-fda-guidance-documents/q2r1-validation-analytical-procedures-text-and-methodology-guidance-industry

17. Guidance for Industry: Process Validation — General Principles and Practices. U.S. Food and Drug Administration: Silver Spring, MD, 2011; https://www.fda.gov/files/drugs/published/Process-Validation–General-Principles-and-Practices.pdf

18. PDA Technical Report 59: Utilization of Statistical Methods for Production Monitoring. (2012). Parenteral Drug Association, Bethesda, MD. https://www.pda.org/bookstore/product-detail/1842-tr-59-utilization-of-statistical-methods

19. Heigl, N., Schmelzer, B., Innerbichler, F., & Shivhare, M. (2021). Statistical quality and process control in Biopharmaceutical manufacturing—Practical issues and remedies. PDA Journal of Pharmaceutical Science and Technology, 75(5), 425-444. https://doi.org/10.5731/pdajpst.2020.011676

20. Nelson, L. S. (1984). The Shewhart control chart—Tests for special causes. Journal of Quality Technology, 16(4), 237-239. https://doi.org/10.1080/00224065.1984.11978921

21. Adhibhatta, S., DiMartino, M., Falcon, R., Haman, E., Legg, K., Payne, R., Pipkins, K., & Zamamiri, A. (2017). Continued process verification (CPV) signal responses in Biopharma. ISPE | International Society for Pharmaceutical Engineering.

Chapter 5: Process Validation: Comprehensive Stability Assessment of Biotechnological Products—Degradation Mechanisms, Statistical Tools, and Regulatory Compliance.

Leveraging Stability Studies: A Strategic Perspective

Physiochemical stability is a critical aspect of biologics manufacturing, directly influencing the quality, safety, and efficacy of the final product. From ancillary solutions to drug substances and drug products, maintaining stability throughout the manufacturing and storage process requires meticulous attention to factors such as temperature, light, shear, container material, and headspace management. This article delves into the key considerations for preserving physiochemical stability at various stages of biologics production, emphasizing the role of proper storage conditions, container selection, and risk mitigation strategies.

Additionally, it explores when small-scale stability data can be leveraged and when full-manufacturing scale data becomes necessary. While small-scale studies are valuable for simulating worst-case scenarios and providing preliminary insights, certain conditions—such as high-risk scenarios, extended storage durations, or regulatory mandates—demand at-scale studies to ensure robust stability evaluations. By understanding and addressing these factors, manufacturers can ensure the integrity of monoclonal antibodies and other biopharmaceuticals, meet regulatory requirements, and uphold the highest standards of product quality.

Ancillary Process Solutions

Ancillary solutions are process-specific reagents or solutions used to facilitate various stages of biologics manufacturing, though they are not part of the final product. These solutions play essential roles in enabling cell culture fermentation, purification, and formulation processes. In the context of monoclonal antibody (mAb) manufacturing, examples of ancillary solutions include buffers used for chromatographic separations (such as phosphate buffer for ion exchange) and media or feed solutions for cell culture. The acceptance of stability data for ancillary solutions, such as cell culture media and buffers, from smaller-scale studies that closely represent commercial manufacturing scale is a recognized practice in the regulatory landscape for biologics [1].

Drug Substance Intermediates

Drug substance intermediates are partially processed forms of the active ingredient (drug substance) that are not yet fully purified or formulated. These intermediates result from earlier stages of purification during biologics manufacturing and require further processing to reach the final drug substance. For mAbs, common examples of DSIs include harvested cell culture fluid (HCCF) after the initial clarification step or a partially purified monoclonal antibody following a protein A capture step but before final polishing and viral filtration. DSIs are typically stored under controlled conditions to maintain their stability and quality until further downstream processing is performed. Manufacturers must identify these intermediates, generate in-house data, and define process limits to ensure their stability within the bounds of the developed process. While small-scale or pilot-plant scale data can be used, manufacturers must compare its suitability by applying the manufacturing-scale process [2].

Drug substance

The drug substance represents the purified and characterized active ingredient intended for formulation into a final product. For mAbs, the drug substance is the highly purified monoclonal antibody obtained after completing key manufacturing steps, including cell culture, harvest and clarification, capture, intermediate and polishing chromatography, and viral clearance filtration. This substance is thoroughly tested for critical quality attributes (CQAs) such as potency, purity, and aggregation. Drug substances are usually stored in liquid or frozen form under tightly controlled conditions until they are ready for conversion into the drug product.

Drug substance (DS) stability cannot be fully leveraged from pilot-scale data for long-term stability purposes. There is always a requirement to include data from at least three at-scale manufacturing batches in the long-term stability program. While pilot-scale data may be acceptable at the time of submission, this is typically a preliminary measure and a commitment must be made to include the first three full-scale manufacturing batches in the long-term stability program post-approval. This ensures that the stability data are representative of the actual manufacturing conditions, processes, and container systems used at the commercial scale. Containers and storage conditions for pilot-scale batches must closely mimic those used at the manufacturing scale for the data to be valid, but they do not replace the need for stability data from full-scale batches [2].

Drug Product

The drug product is the final formulated and packaged form of the biologic, ready for administration to patients. For mAbs, this involves formulating the drug substance with excipients such as stabilizers and buffers to ensure its stability and delivery. After formulation, the product undergoes sterile filtration and is aseptically filled into its final container, which may be vials, syringes, or cartridges. The drug product is then packaged and labeled for distribution. Stringent quality control testing, including sterility, potency, and appearance evaluations, ensures the product meets all regulatory standards before it reaches patients.

Although pilot-scale stability data may be included in the submission, it must be accompanied by a commitment to place the first three manufacturing-scale batches into a long-term stability program post-approval [2].

Impact of Storage Container Properties on the Physiochemical Stability of Monoclonal Antibodies and Proteins

The EMA identifies several common instability issues in therapeutic proteins, including deamidation (hydrolysis of asparagine and glutamine side chains), oxidation of residues such as methionine, histidine, cysteine, tyrosine, and tryptophan, aggregation (covalent or noncovalent association of monomers or native multimers), and glycoprotein instability, particularly the hydrolysis of sialic acid residues. The stability of drug products varies depending on their specific characteristics and formulation types. Table 1 summarizes the storage container parameters commonly assessed for protein stability to determine the suitability of using pilot- or bench-scale data to represent manufacturing-scale conditions [3].

Parameter	Impact on Quality Attributes
Temperature	Maintaining precise storage temperatures is critical for preventing protein denaturation, aggregation, or loss of activity. Deviations can accelerate chemical degradation, such as deamidation or oxidation, reducing the monoclonal antibody's efficacy and shelf life. Temperature-controlled storage and controlled rate of temperature change are considered negligible risks [4].
Light	mAbs are sensitive to photo-degradation, which can cause oxidation of methionine residues and other chemical modifications, leading to compromised structural integrity and therapeutic efficacy. Opaque containers are considered a negligible risk [5].
Shear	Shear from mixing disrupts protein structures, potentially causing degradation, aggregation and increased subvisible particles [4]. For intermediates and drug substances, matching the shear surrogate operating parameters like power by volume or impeller tip speed are considered negligible risks.
Container Material	The choice of container material is crucial as plastics can lead to protein adsorption and the introduction of leachable, while glass containers pose risks of delamination, which can release subvisible particles into the formulation [6]. To enhance the flexibility of stability testing, manufacturers can leverage small stainless-steel containers or stainless-steel stability bottles. These options allow for precise simulation of manufacturing-scale storage conditions while minimizing resource use.
Headspace Gassing	The presence of oxygen in the headspace of containers is a critical factor that can accelerate the oxidative degradation of proteins, leading to a loss of pH stability and overall product efficacy. This phenomenon is particularly significant in biopharmaceutical formulations, where proteins are highly sensitive to oxidative stress [7]. Furthermore, the use of inert gases such as nitrogen has been shown to mitigate oxidative stress, thereby preserving the integrity of protein formulations. This is supported by studies indicating that replacing oxygen with inert gases can significantly enhance the stability of biopharmaceuticals by reducing the rate of oxidation and

Parameter	Impact on Quality Attributes
	subsequent degradation, although specific studies directly addressing this claim were not identified in the provided references [8]. Therefore, effective management of headspace in biopharmaceutical containers is essential for maintaining protein stability and ensuring product quality.
Headspace Volume in small containers like Vials	For drug products, the amount of headspace in vials plays a role not only in cavitation phenomena but also in protein stability and potential aggregation [9]. This suggests that optimizing headspace volume is vital for maintaining the stability of protein formulations, as excessive headspace can lead to increased oxidative stress, and insufficient headspace can create pressure conditions that may promote aggregation.
Container Closure	Poor seals lead to contamination, pH instability, and oxidation due to oxygen/moisture ingress [10].

Conclusion: Transforming Stability Evaluations for Tomorrow

To optimize stability assessments, manufacturers should leverage small-scale studies to simulate worst-case scenarios, including extreme storage durations, temperature ranges, and stress conditions when not mandated by regulatory agencies [3]. This approach reduces the need for at-scale studies while ensuring risks are addressed. At-scale studies should be reserved for high-risk scenarios or cases mandated by regulatory agencies. This strategy ensures resource efficiency while maintaining compliance and supporting high-quality biologics production data utilization while maintaining product quality and regulatory compliance.

References

1. Biophorum. (2021, May 5). Justification of small-scale models: An industry perspective. Retrieved from https://www.biophorum.com/download/justification-of-small-scale-models-an-industry-perspective/

2. U.S. Food and Drug Administration. (2007). Guidance for industry: Q1A(R2) stability testing of new drug substances and products. Retrieved from https://www.fda.gov/media/71707/download

3. G. Jimenez, Brake B. ICH Q5C Stability Testing of Biotechnological/Biological Products. EMA Training for ASEAN, 30–31 May 2011. https://admin.ich.org/sites/default/files/inline-files/SESSION_Ia_ICH_Q5C.pdf

4. Nayak, P., Goode, M., Chang, D. P., & Rajagopal, K. (2020). Ectoine and hydroxyectoine stabilize antibodies in spray-dried formulations at elevated temperature and during a freeze/thaw process. Molecular Pharmaceutics, 17(9), 3291-3297. https://doi.org/10.1021/acs.molpharmaceut.0c00395

5. Shah, D. D., Zhang, J., Maity, H., & Mallela, K. M. G. (2018). Effect of photo-degradation on the structure, stability, aggregation, and function of an IgG1 monoclonal antibody. International journal of pharmaceutics, 547(1-2), 438–449. https://doi.org/10.1016/j.ijpharm.2018.06.007

6. Bee, J. S., Randolph, T. W., Carpenter, J. F., Bishop, S. M., & Dimitrova, M. N. (2011). Effects of surfaces and leachables on the stability of biopharmaceuticals. Journal of Pharmaceutical Sciences, 100(10), 4158–4170. https://doi.org/10.1002/jps.22597

7. Zheng, K., Ren, D., Wang, Y. J., Lilyestrom, W., Scherer, T., Hong, J. K. Y., & Ji, J. A. (2021). Monoclonal Antibody Aggregation Associated with Free Radical Induced Oxidation. International journal of molecular sciences, 22(8), 3952. https://doi.org/10.3390/ijms22083952

8. United States Pharmacopeia. (2023). General Chapter: ⟨1059⟩ Excipient Performance. In USP-NF. Rockville, MD: United States Pharmacopeia. https://doi.org/10.31003/USPNF_M2312_05_01

9. Valotta Rodrigues, R., Puryear, M., Sederstrom, D., & Lengsfeld, C. S. (2019). Parameters Influencing Cavitation Within Vials Subjected to Drop Shock. Scientific reports, 9(1), 19210. https://doi.org/10.1038/s41598-019-55668-9

10. Zeng, Q. (2021, September/October). Safeguarding vial container closure integrity: A systematic approach. Pharmaceutical Engineering. Retrieved from https://ispe.org/pharmaceutical-engineering/september-october-2021/safeguarding-vial-container-closure-integrity

Chapter 6: Comprehensive Risk Assessment and Classification of Raw Materials in Biologics Manufacturing

Introduction

Stability testing is a fundamental component of pharmaceutical and biotechnological product development, ensuring that a product's quality, safety, and efficacy are maintained throughout its shelf life. This critical process evaluates how environmental factors, such as temperature, humidity, and light, affect the product over time, enabling the establishment of robust shelf life and storage conditions. Stability studies also support regulatory submissions by providing comprehensive data to demonstrate the consistency and reliability of the product under various conditions. A key focus of stability assessments is understanding degradation mechanisms, including aggregation, oxidation, and chemical modifications, which can impact product integrity. Statistical approaches, such as regression analysis and Analysis of Covariance (ANCOVA), play an essential role in modeling degradation trends and ensuring consistency across batches. These methodologies enable precise determination of expiration dates and retest periods, aligning with regulatory expectations.

The application of tools like the Arrhenius equation allows for long-term stability predictions using accelerated data, offering insights into product behavior at typical storage conditions without waiting for real-time data. By integrating advanced analytical techniques, statistical rigor, and predictive models, stability testing provides a robust framework to mitigate risks, ensure product quality, and meet regulatory requirements throughout the product lifecycle.

Stability Studies and Their Integration Across Clinical Trial Phases and Manufacturing.

Stability studies are critical for determining a product's shelf life and storage requirements, as well as understanding how environmental factors such as temperature, humidity, and light affect product quality [1]. These studies are typically categorized into three types based on the conditions applied: long-term, intermediate, and accelerated stability studies.

The stability evaluation process is often divided into three phases based on the product life cycle:

- Phase I, initial formulation stability, is evaluated through short-term accelerated studies designed to identify potential degradation pathways. These studies often subject the mAb to stress conditions, such as 40°C/75% RH for 1–3 months, to simulate extreme environments and accelerate degradation [2]. Analytical testing in this phase includes quantification of the mAb concentration using high-performance liquid chromatography (HPLC-UV) and the assessment of purity via size-exclusion chromatography (SEC). Additional tests, such as visual inspection for physical changes like color, clarity, or particulate formation, provide further insights [4]. Advanced methods such as liquid chromatography-mass spectrometry (LC-MS) are utilized to identify chemical modifications, including oxidation, deamidation, and fragmentation. Data from Phase I inform the selection of buffer formulations and provide a foundational understanding of the mAb's stability under stress.
- Phase II involves a more comprehensive assessment of stability under intermediate and long-term storage conditions. For example, studies may be conducted at 25°C/60% RH and 5°C for durations of 6–12 months [1]. During this phase, analytical methods are expanded to include evaluations of charge variants using ion-exchange chromatography (IEX) and assessments of protein structure through techniques such as differential scanning calorimetry (DSC) or circular dichroism (CD) spectroscopy [5]. These techniques confirm the thermal stability and secondary structure integrity of the mAb over time. Additionally, Phase II explores the stability of mAb formulations in various container closure systems, such as glass vials or prefilled syringes, under simulated shipping conditions, including freeze-thaw and agitation stress. This phase ensures the stability of the product under real-world conditions while verifying the compatibility of the mAb with packaging materials.
- Phase III represents the most extensive phase of stability testing, supporting regulatory submissions and market authorization. Long-term stability studies are conducted across multiple batches of the mAb, typically over its entire proposed shelf life (e.g., 2–3 years at 5°C) [8]. These studies involve rigorous testing to confirm potency through cell-based bioassays, ensuring that the biological activity of the mAb remains consistent

throughout storage. Degradation products, such as aggregates, fragments, and chemical modifications like glycation or carbamylation, are quantified to evaluate potential impacts on efficacy and safety [9]. Shelf-life modeling based on Phase III data establishes expiration dates and recommended storage conditions [3]. For instance, demonstrating consistent stability at 5°C over two years across three production batches can justify a shelf-life claim of 24 months under refrigerated conditions.

This phased approach ensures a comprehensive understanding of mAb stability from early development through commercialization. By systematically addressing degradation pathways, storage compatibility, and long-term viability, stability studies form a cornerstone of regulatory compliance and commercial success for monoclonal antibody therapeutics [1, 10].

The scale of manufacturing also evolves through the clinical phases. Phase I typically relies on early-stage process development batches, often produced at a small scale in the laboratory, to test the drug in a limited patient population [11]. By Phase II, larger-scale tech transfer batches are utilized as the process scales up to support broader clinical studies [9]. In Phase III, process performance qualification (PPQ) batches are manufactured to support pivotal clinical trials, demonstrating the process's readiness for commercialization and regulatory submission [12]. Stability studies during these stages provide essential data to ensure the product's quality, safety, and efficacy throughout its lifecycle [8].

Stability Study Requirements for Change in Technology or Site Transfer in Drug Substances

FDA's Guidance for Industry: Changes to an approved NDA or ANDA (2004), recommends when transitioning the manufacturing site for a drug substance, stability studies are essential to confirm that the change does not significantly impact the stability of the product. These studies ensure the drug substance maintains its quality, potency, and safety throughout its shelf life [13]. The new stability studies are conducted at the new site, including comparative evaluations with data from the original site to detect any potential differences in the stability profile. Both long-term and accelerated stability studies are usually required to demonstrate that the relocation of manufacturing does not adversely affect the drug substance. FDA's Revised proposal on site-specific stability data (1994) states If sufficient primary stability data are available, 3 months of accelerated and long-term data on one batch may suffice. However, if primary data are insufficient, stability studies on three batches are generally required, along with a standard stability commitment to monitor the product over its intended shelf life [14].

Table 1: Summary of Stability Studies and Their Integration Across Clinical Trial Phases and Manufacturing Scales.

Phase	Description	Batch Scale
Phase I	Initial formulation stability studies focus on identifying degradation pathways through short-term accelerated studies (e.g., 40°C/75% RH for 1–3 months). These studies simulate stress conditions to evaluate product stability.	Small-scale lab batches are used for initial patient testing.
Phase II	Comprehensive stability assessment under intermediate and long-term storage conditions (e.g., 25°C/60% RH and 5°C for 6–12 months). This phase also evaluates container closure systems and real-world stress conditions like freeze-thaw and agitation.	Larger-scale tech transfer batches to support broader clinical studies.
Phase III	Full-scale long-term stability studies are performed to support regulatory submissions and establish shelf life. These studies evaluate multiple production batches under real-world conditions, ensuring efficacy and safety throughout the	PPQ batches for pivotal clinical trials, demonstrating process readiness for commercialization.

Phase	Description	Batch Scale
	proposed shelf life (e.g., 2–3 years at 5°C).	

Selection of Batches

Stability studies should include at least three batches of drug substances or drug products. For bulk materials stored prior to formulation, a minimum of six months of stability data is required for requested storage periods exceeding this duration. Pilot-scale batches may be utilized initially, with a commitment to evaluate manufacturing-scale batches post-approval. The batches selected for stability studies must represent the quality of material used in preclinical and clinical studies. For final container products, data should include different bulk material batches where possible, ensuring robust stability evaluation [1]. Moreover, ICH Q1A offers guidance on the selection of stability batches. The process validation lifecycle strategy and the regulatory requirements of the target registration jurisdiction determine the number of batches selected for stability monitoring. Stability monitoring should include all batches manufactured during PPQ unless a compelling business justification exists for monitoring only a subset of these batches [1,15].

Frequency of Testing Points

In long-term stability studies, the testing frequency must adequately establish the drug product's stability profile. For products with a proposed shelf life of at least 12 months, testing at the long-term storage condition should occur every three months during the first year, every six months in the second year, and annually thereafter throughout the shelf life. For accelerated storage conditions, a minimum of three-time points—initial, intermediate, and final (e.g., 0, 3, and 6 months)—should be included in a six-month study. If development data suggest that accelerated testing results may approach significant change criteria, testing should be intensified by adding a fourth-time point or increasing sample testing at the final time point.

When intermediate storage condition testing is required due to significant changes observed at the accelerated storage condition, a 12-month study with at least four-time points—initial, intermediate, and final (e.g., 0, 6, 9, and 12 months)—is recommended. Reduced testing designs, such as matrixing or bracketing, may be employed to decrease the testing frequency or omit specific factor combinations, provided these approaches are scientifically justified [1].

Replicates of samples at given Testing time Points

When feasible, replicating testing at specific time points can provide statistical advantages by improving the precision of slope estimates. Chow (2007) reports replication is particularly valuable at the beginning and end of the study timeline, as it helps mitigate the influence of outlier observations at high-leverage time points. Such outliers could disproportionately affect slope calculations, especially at later stages when degradation is expected [16]. If replicating samples at certain time points is not possible, closely spaced sampling at the beginning and end of the study can enhance the robustness of slope estimates. For instance, for a recommended storage condition with a 24-month shelf life, sampling could be scheduled at 20 and 22 months. Similarly, in accelerated stability studies with a 3-month timeline, additional testing could be performed at intervals such as 0.25, 0.5, 2.5, and 2.75 months [15].

Bracketing and Matrixing Approaches in Stability Studies

Bracketing involves testing the "extreme" combinations of factors, such as the lowest and highest storage temperatures or fill volumes, at all-time points, assuming the stability of intermediate conditions falls within the range established by the extremes. For example, in a drug product stored at three temperatures (T1, T2, and T3) and three fill volumes (V1, V2, and V3), a bracketing design that tests only the two extreme fill volumes (V1 and V3) would generate six data sets representing the 3x2 temperature-volume combinations. Researchers analyze these data sets to estimate shelf life while assessing the assumption that intermediate temperatures or fill volumes exhibit stability similar to the extremes. If the analysis reveals that the stability at extreme temperatures or fill volumes differs, the intermediate conditions are considered no more stable than the least stable extreme. For instance, if V1 is less stable than V3, the shelf life for V2 should not exceed that of V1, and interpolation between V1 and V3 is avoided [17].

Matrixing, by contrast, tests a subset of all possible factor combinations at each time point, ensuring that the entire set of combinations is evaluated throughout the study. Coffey (2020) highlights that matrixing is particularly suitable for small molecules, as it assumes a high level of product knowledge, as outlined in ICH Q5C [15]. This article does not address matrixing in the context of large molecules due to its limited applicability. While matrixing reduces the testing burden by focusing on a representative subset, it relies heavily on robust product understanding to ensure stability assumptions across untested combinations are valid.

Stability-Indicating Profile

No single assay can fully characterize the stability of biotechnological products. Manufacturers must develop a stability-indicating profile that detects changes in identity, purity, and potency. Validated methods tailored to the product-specific attributes are critical. These profiles should document degradation pathways, enabling the establishment of acceptable limits for product degradation [18]. Quality attributes typically assessed in biologics protein manufacturing are summarized in Table 2.

Table 2: Quality Attributes assessed in Biologics DS stability study.

Attribute	Typical Degradation Pathways	References
Identity	Deamidation, isomerization, fragmentation	[19, 20]
Purity	Aggregation, oxidation, glycation	[18, 21]
Potency	Aggregation, glycosylation changes, loss of conformational stability	[22, 23]

Mechanisms and Kinetics of Protein Degradation

Protein degradation in biotechnological products involves various pathways, each driven by specific mechanisms and following characteristic kinetics. Understanding these pathways is critical for modeling the degradation rate to establish shelf life. Table 3 is a comprehensive overview of key degradation mechanisms and their kinetics.

Table 3: Comprehensive overview of key degradation mechanisms and their kinetics.

Degradation Pathway	Mechanism	Kinetics	References
Protein Aggregation	Formation of dimers, oligomers, or insoluble aggregates driven by hydrophobic interactions, hydrogen bonding, or stress (e.g., shear, heat).	Sigmoidal kinetics: lag phase followed by growth phase (first-order).	[21, 24]
Protein Oxidation	Modifications of amino acid side chains (e.g., methionine, cysteine) by reactive oxygen species (ROS).	Pseudo-first-order kinetics when the oxidant is in excess; second-order kinetics for equimolar reactants.	[25, 26]
Protein Deamidation	Hydrolysis of asparagine (Asn) or glutamine (Gln) residues to aspartic acid (Asp), isoaspartic acid (isoAsp), or glutamic acid (Glu); influenced by temperature, pH, and buffers.	First-order kinetics with rates increasing exponentially with temperature (Arrhenius behavior).	[27, 28]
Protein Reduction	Cleavage of disulfide bonds to form free thiol groups using reducing agents like DTT or beta-mercaptoethanol.	Pseudo-first-order kinetics when the reducing agent is in excess; second-order kinetics for equimolar reactants.	[29,30]
Changes in Glycosylation	Alterations are caused by enzymatic activity or environmental factors, including hydrolysis of glycosidic bonds or	First-order kinetics for hydrolytic or enzymatic processes; pseudo-first-order kinetics for reactions	[31, 32]

Degradation Pathway	Mechanism	Kinetics	References
	oxidation of sugar residues.	with limiting reactants.	
Protein Glycation	Non-enzymatic reaction of reducing sugars with amino groups in proteins, forming advanced glycation end products (AGEs).	First-order or pseudo-first-order kinetics depending on sugar concentration.	[33,35]

This integrated framework of degradation mechanisms and kinetics serves as a foundational reference for evaluating and establishing product stability shelf-life period. Different degradation pathway follows different orders of reaction rate. Integrated form and linear regression equation for different orders of reaction rate shown in Table 4 [36].

Table 4: Oder of Reactions and Regression Models

Order	Rate Law	Integrated Form	Linear Equation Form
Pseudo-First-Order	$\frac{d[A]}{dt} = -k[A]$	$[A] = [A]_0 e^{-kt}$	$\ln[A] = \ln[A]_0 - kt$
First-Order	$\frac{d[A]}{dt} = -k[A]$	$[A] = [A]_0 e^{-kt}$	$\ln[A] = \ln[A]_0 - kt$

Second-Order	$\frac{d[A]}{dt} = -k[A]^2$	$\frac{1}{[A]} = \frac{1}{[A]_0} + kt$	$\frac{1}{[A]} = \frac{1}{[A]_0} + kt$

Statistical Approach to Shelf-Life Determination: Applying ICH Q1(E) Guidelines for Robust Pharmaceutical Stability Assessment

In accordance with ICH Q1(E) guidelines, the determination of retest periods or shelf lives for pharmaceutical products should be based on a conservative approach utilizing the 95% confidence interval of the regression line rather than relying solely on the regression line itself. This ensures an added safety margin to account for variability, thereby safeguarding product quality and patient safety. Shelf lives or retest periods should initially be calculated for individual batches using batch-specific intercepts and slopes, pooled mean square error, and the 95% confidence limit [34].

If all batches independently support the proposed retest period or shelf life, the product is deemed compliant. However, if one or more batches fail to meet the proposed retest period or shelf life, poolability tests may be employed to determine whether data from these batches can be combined. Pooling involves assessing the consistency of slopes across batches and, if common slopes are established, recalculating shelf lives using batch-specific intercepts while considering pooled variability. When pooling reveals that the recalculated retest periods exceed the proposed period, further testing of intercepts for poolability may not be necessary. This conservative approach ensures that shelf lives are determined with a robust margin of safety, minimizing the risk of overestimating stability while adhering to regulatory requirements. The emphasis on confidence intervals and the iterative evaluation of batch data exemplifies a methodologically rigorous and patient-centric approach to pharmaceutical stability assessment [1].

Which Interval is Appropriate for Stability Studies: Confidence or Tolerance?

In stability studies, mean confidence intervals define the range for the true mean of stability data, and tolerance intervals predict the range where a specified proportion of the population will fall, accounting for variability. The ICH Q1E guidelines recommend using regression analysis with mean confidence intervals to determine shelf life, ensuring the product remains within specifications over time. Researchers often apply tolerance intervals as a more conservative approach [34], as these address variability and ensure a defined proportion of future batches meet specifications. While not explicitly required by ICH, tolerance intervals are particularly valuable for high-risk products or cases with significant variability [15]. Table 5 below provides concise steps for performing regression analysis in JMP, including entering data, fitting the model, and saving predicted values and confidence intervals.

Table 5: Step by step procedure to generate confidence intervals on regression line using JMP.

Step	Action	Result
Step 1	Open JMP and create a new data table. Enter columns for Time (X) and Observed (Y).	Your raw data is entered into JMP.
Step 2	Go to Analyze > Fit Y by X, assign Time to X and Observed to Y, then click OK.	Regression analysis is performed, and the scatterplot with the regression line is displayed.
Step 3	Click the red triangle next to the regression title. Select Save Columns > Predicted Values.	A new column with predicted values is added to the data table.
Step 5	Click the red triangle and select Save Columns > Mean Confidence Limits.	Two new columns, Lower Mean CI and Upper Mean CI, are added for the **Mean Confidence Interval**.

Table 6 outlines a step-by-step guide for using JMP to perform regression analysis and calculate tolerance intervals. This process involves preparing the data, fitting a regression model, and calculating key statistical measures like residuals, residual standard error, and standard error of prediction.

Additionally, it provides instructions for computing the tolerance bounds, which include the upper and lower limits for a specified confidence level and proportion of the population. Each step includes the necessary actions and the corresponding results, making it a practical roadmap for implementing the analysis in JMP. Table 6 summarizes the steps involved in the generation of the Tolerance interval on the regression line using JMP.

Table 6: Step-by-step procedure to generate Tolerance intervals on regression line using JMP.

Step	Action and Result
Step 1: Enter Data	Open JMP and create a new data table. Enter two columns: **Time (X)** (Independent variable) and **Observed (Y)** (Dependent variable/response).
Step 2: Fit the Model	Go to Analyze > Fit Y by X, assign **Y** (Observed) as the response and **X** (Time) as the factor, then click OK to generate the regression model and scatterplot.
Step 3: Predicted Values	Click the red triangle next to the regression title and select Save Columns > Predicted Values. A new column with predicted values
Step 4: Residuals	From the same red triangle menu, select Save Columns > Residuals. A new column with residuals will be added to the table.
Step 5: Residual Sum of Squares (RSS)	Create a column for Residual Sum of Squared = $(\text{Residual})^2$
Step 6: Residual Standard Error (s)	Create a column for $$s = \sqrt{\left(\frac{\sum RSS}{n}\right)}$$
Step 7, Calculate (k) Factor for Tolerance Intervals	Create a column for (k), Default α =0.05, and population proportion (p)=0.99. $$k = t_{\frac{\alpha}{2},n-1} \times z_p \times \sqrt{1 + \frac{1}{n} + \frac{\chi^2_{p,n-2}}{n-2}}$$
Step 8, Calculate Standard	Create a column for,

Step	Action and Result
Error of Prediction, SE(X)	$SE(X) = s.\sqrt{\frac{1}{n} + \frac{(X_i - X_{avg})^2}{\sum(X_i - X_{avg})^2}}$
Step 9: Calculate the Upper and Lower Tolerance Bounds	$TB = Y \pm k.SE(X)$

Assessing Poolability in Stability Studies

In pharmaceutical stability studies, assessing the poolability of data from different lots is crucial when multiple batches are involved in determining a product's shelf life or retest period. Poolability assessments are particularly important when variability between lots could affect the interpretation of stability data. This evaluation is necessary in scenarios such as establishing a common shelf life or retest period, where pooling helps determine if a single model can represent all batches. Regulatory compliance also drives the need for robust justification of pooled data to ensure product safety and quality [1]. Additionally, poolability assessments are essential when there is significant variability in manufacturing or storage conditions between lots to ensure that these differences do not compromise the stability conclusions. Pooling may also be required if individual lots lack sufficient data points to establish stability trends independently. Furthermore, statistical consistency among batches is a prerequisite for valid pooling, as it ensures all lots exhibit similar degradation trends over time.

ICH Q1E recommends Analysis of Covariance (ANCOVA) as a statistical method used to assess whether stability data from different lots can be pooled [34]. It evaluates the main effects, including the impact of time, by testing overall trends in stability data over time and the effect of batches by examining differences in initial stability levels between lots. Additionally, ANCOVA assesses the interaction effect between time and batch (Time*Batch) to determine whether the slopes, which represent degradation rates, are consistent across lots. A significant interaction effect, indicated by a p-value less than 0.05, suggests non-poolability, as it reveals inconsistent slopes among the batches [38]. Table 7 shows the step by step methodology to perform ANCOVA using JMP.

Table 7: Steps to Perform ANCOVA in JMP	
Step 1: Prepare Your Data	Organize your data in a spreadsheet-like format with the following columns: - Batch: Categorical variable (e.g., A, B, C). - Time: Continuous variable (e.g., 1, 2, 3, etc.). - Response: Observed values (e.g., concentration or stability data).
Step 3: Run ANCOVA	1. Open JMP and import your dataset. 2. Go to the Analyze menu and select Fit Model. 3. In the Fit Model window: - Drag Response to the Y (Response) box. - Drag Time and Batch to the Construct Model Effects box. - Add Time*Batch to the model effects to test for interaction. 4. Click Run.
Step 4: Interpret Results	- Main Effects: Check if the p-values for Time and Batch are significant to confirm the main effects. - Interaction Effect (Time*Batch): If the p-value for the interaction effect is < 0.05, it indicates significant differences in slopes across batches, meaning the data are not poolable. If the interaction effect is insignificant, it suggests the data can be pooled for further analysis.

For the purpose of illustrating the concepts of confidence intervals and tolerance intervals on a regression line, the data published by Coffey and Yang (Eds., 2018) is utilized, as shown in Figure 1 [15]. The methodologies outlined in Tables 5 and 6 are applied to generate both the confidence and tolerance intervals. This approach visually demonstrates the differences between the two intervals and highlights how the tolerance interval is more conservative compared to the confidence interval. The tolerance interval accounts for the uncertainty arising from the limited sample size, thereby providing a broader range to accommodate potential variability in future observations.

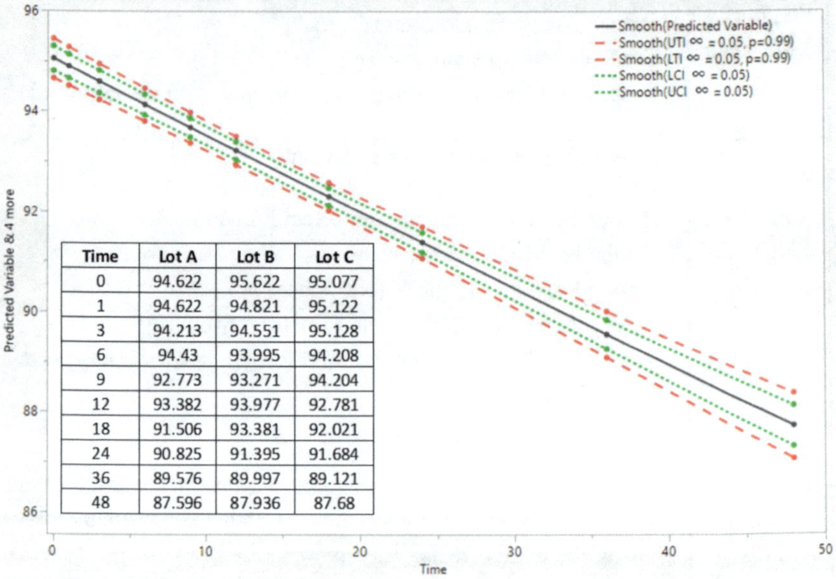

Time	Lot A	Lot B	Lot C
0	94.622	95.622	95.077
1	94.622	94.821	95.122
3	94.213	94.551	95.128
6	94.43	93.995	94.208
9	92.773	93.271	94.204
12	93.382	93.977	92.781
18	91.506	93.381	92.021
24	90.825	91.395	91.684
36	89.576	89.997	89.121
48	87.596	87.936	87.68

Extending Product Shelf Life Using Accelerated Stability Studies: A Structured Approach

Extending the shelf life of a pharmaceutical product based on accelerated stability studies requires robust scientific evidence demonstrating that the product maintains its quality, potency, and safety under stress conditions. These conditions simulate longer-term storage and provide a predictive framework for determining product stability. A systematic approach is essential to justify shelf-life extensions and meet regulatory expectations [1, 39].

The first step involves conducting accelerated stability studies under stress conditions such as elevated temperature and humidity, following guidelines like ICH Q1A(R2) [1, 34]. Typical conditions for most drug products include 40°C/75% RH, while biologics may require tailored stress conditions. During these studies, manufacturers monitor critical quality attributes, including assay, impurities, potency, and physical appearance, over a shorter duration (e.g., 3–6 months) to identify degradation patterns [5].

Data analysis is critical for identifying trends in degradation. Statistical methods, such as regression analysis, help project product stability under normal storage conditions [3]. If real-time stability data are available, researchers can correlate these with accelerated data to validate that degradation mechanisms are consistent across different conditions. This ensures that predictions based on accelerated studies accurately reflect long-term stability [4].

Manufacturers often use the Arrhenius equation or similar models to extrapolate long-term stability from accelerated data. The Arrhenius equation predicts the effect of temperature on the degradation rate, allowing for the estimation of shelf life. To ensure confidence in these projections, statistical validation, including confidence intervals, is necessary [11]. Regulatory submissions seeking shelf-life extensions must include both accelerated and real-time stability data supported by thorough statistical analyses and justifications [1, 34]. Compliance with ICH guidelines, such as Q1E, ensures adherence to regulatory standards for data pooling and retest period extrapolation. Authorities may grant shelf-life extensions if the data and modeling demonstrate scientific validity [8].

However, regulatory limits constrain the extent of shelf-life extensions. These cannot exceed twice the duration of the original stability studies or extend more than 12 months beyond available real-time data, whichever is shorter [34]. Manufacturers must also commit to ongoing real-time stability studies to confirm the extended shelf life and report any unexpected findings, such as out-of-specification results, to regulatory authorities promptly [39]. Consistency between accelerated and real-time degradation mechanisms is paramount, as is the statistical validation of extrapolated data. Ensuring regulatory compliance through alignment with regional guidelines, including those from the FDA, EMA, and ICH, is critical to a successful shelf-life extension. By integrating accelerated and real-time stability data with statistical modeling, manufacturers can scientifically justify shelf-life extensions. This approach not only ensures product quality and safety but also supports regulatory compliance and market success [1, 11].

Predicting Long-Term Stability from Accelerated Stability Data Using the Arrhenius Equation

The Arrhenius equation, as shown in Equation 1, describes the relationship between temperature and the rate of chemical reactions:

$$k = Ae^{-\left(\frac{E_a}{R.T}\right)} \quad \text{Eq (1)}$$

Where: k: Reaction rate constant (units/month), A: Frequency factor (pre-exponential constant), Ea: Activation energy (J/mol), R: Universal gas constant (8.314 J/mol\K) and T: Absolute temperature (K). In the actual study, the degradation rate constants (k) at 25°C and 40°C were determined experimentally, and the activation energy (Ea) was calculated using a linear regression approach.

To illustrate the methodology described in this study, the data presented in Figure 2 was recreated from the previously published work by Kuzman et al., 2021 [40]. Table 8 demonstrates the methodology to predict the log-term stability data from accelerated stability data using the Arrhenius equation.

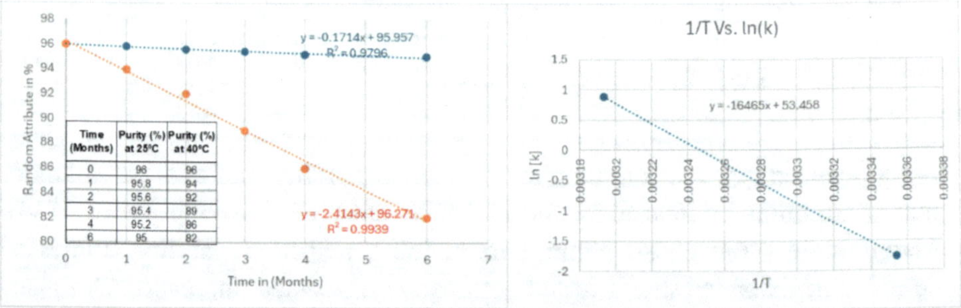

Time (Months)	Purity (%) at 25°C	Purity (%) at 40°C
0	96	96
1	95.8	94
2	95.6	92
3	95.4	89
4	95.2	86
6	95	82

Table 8: Illustrative Calculation Predicting Long-Term Stability from Accelerated Stability Data Using the Arrhenius Equation

Step 1: Calculation of Activation Energy. To apply the Arrhenius equation, experimental data were used to calculate degradation rate constants ("k") at two temperatures, as shown in Figure 2A: • At T = 25 + 273.15 = 298.15 K, k = 0.1714 units/month. • At T = 40 + 273.15 = 313.15 K, k = 2.4143 units/month. A linear regression plot of "ln(k)" versus "1/T" was generated, as shown in Figure 2B, resulting in a slope of -16,455.5 K. The slope was used to calculate the activation energy ("E_a"): E_a = -slope × R = 16,465 × 8.314 = 136,890 J/mol.
Step 2. Calculation of degradation at rate. To predict the degradation rate constant ("k") at 5°C (T = 278.15 K), the Arrhenius equation was rearranged to: $$\ln(k) = \ln(A) - \left(\frac{E_a}{R.T}\right)$$ Substituting the values: $$\ln(k) = \ln(A) - \left(\frac{136{,}890}{8.314 \times 278.15}\right)$$ From Figure 2B, Using the regression intercept, ln(A) = 53.46 $$\ln(k) = 53.46 - \left(\frac{136{,}890}{8.314 \times 278.15}\right) = -5.7$$ Exponentiating: k = exp (-0.57) ≈ 0.003 units/month.
Step 3: Calculate the predicted Shelf life at target temperature. The shelf life of the product was calculated as the time required for its purity to decrease from 96% (initial) to 95% (acceptable limit). Using the formula: t = ("Initial Purity" - "Final Purity") / k, Substituting the values: t = (96 - 95) / 0.0032 = 5 / 0.003 ≈ 55.5 months. Converting months to years:

t = 55.5 / 12 ≈ 4.6 years.

The application of the Arrhenius equation predicted a degradation rate constant ("k") of 0.003 units/month at 5°C, corresponding to a shelf life of approximately 55.5 months (4.6 years). This example highlights the utility of the Arrhenius model for predicting long-term stability based on accelerated stability data, providing a robust tool for pharmaceutical shelf-life estimation.

Mean Kinetic Temperature (MKT)

MKT is a calculated value used in pharmaceutical stability studies to represent the cumulative thermal stress under different temperatures experienced by a product over time. It is defined as the single temperature at which the total degradation experienced would be equivalent to the degradation over a range of temperatures. MKT is particularly useful for assessing the impact of temperature fluctuations during storage and transportation. The British Medicines Authority (MHRA) advises: "Do not use Mean Kinetic Temperature (MKT) to compensate for inadequate temperature control in storage facilities. Apply it only in cases where temperature control is generally reliable, but occasional excursions occur". Per USP <1079.2>, MKT is calculated using the Arrhenius equation as shown in Equation-2 [41], incorporating factors such as activation energy (Ea), the gas constant (R), absolute temperature (Ti), and the duration of exposure (ti). Below is a sample calculation illustrating how MKT is derived using temperature readings over 20 days with specified time intervals, assuming Ea = 136,890 J/mol from the previous example.

$$MKT = \frac{E_a/_R}{ln\left(\frac{\sum\left(e^{\frac{-E_a}{R.T_i}}.t_i\right)}{\sum t_i}\right)} \qquad \text{Eq (2)}$$

Table 9: Calculation of logarithmic term in MKT Equation

Interval	Temp (°C)	Temp (K)	(-Ea) /(RT)	Time, t (Days)	[(-Ea) /(RT)]× t
T1	25	298	1.01E-24	10	1.01E-23
T2	30	303	2.51E-24	5	1.26E-23
T3	35	308	6.08E-24	3	1.82E-23
T4	40	313	1.43E-23	2	2.85E-23
			Total	20	6.9E-23

$$MKT = \frac{136{,}890/8.314}{ln\left(\frac{6.9E-23}{20}\right)} = 304.8\ °K \approx 31.65℃ \qquad \text{Eq (2)}$$

Conclusion

The stability testing of biotechnological products integrates an understanding of degradation mechanisms, storage conditions, and statistical evaluation to ensure product quality over time. Key considerations such as batch selection, testing frequency, and stability-indicating assays form the foundation of these studies. Statistical methods, including linear regression and ANCOVA, provide critical insights into the stability profiles of pharmaceutical products and enable informed decisions about pooling data from different batches. These analyses not only ensure compliance with regulatory guidelines but also safeguard patient safety by minimizing variability and maintaining robust product quality. By applying scientifically rigorous approaches, manufacturers can confidently establish shelf lives, optimize formulations, and maintain the integrity of biopharmaceutical products throughout their lifecycle.

References

1. International Conference on Harmonisation (ICH). (2003). Stability testing of new drug substances and products Q1A(R2). Retrieved from https://database.ich.org/sites/default/files/Q1A%28R2%29%20Guideline.pdf
2. World Health Organization (WHO). (2009). Stability Testing of Active Pharmaceutical Ingredients and Finished Pharmaceutical Products. https://cdn.who.int/media/docs/default-source/medicines/norms-and-standards/guidelines/regulatory-standards/trs953-annex2-appendix1-stability-conditions-table-2018.pdf?sfvrsn=74032aec_12&download=true
3. Waterman, K. C., & Adami, R. C. (2005). Accelerated aging: Prediction of chemical stability of pharmaceuticals. International Journal of Pharmaceutics, 293(1-2), 101-125. https://doi.org/10.1016/j.ijpharm.2004.12.013
4. Ahuja, S., & Scypinski, S. (Eds.). (2001). Handbook of modern pharmaceutical analysis. Academic Press.
5. Blessy, M., Patel, R. D., Prajapati, P. N., & Agrawal, Y. K. (2014). Development of forced degradation and stability indicating studies of drugs-A review. Journal of pharmaceutical analysis, 4(3), 159–165. https://doi.org/10.1016/j.jpha.2013.09.003
6. Hawe, A., Sutter, M., & Jiskoot, W. (2008). Extrinsic particle characterization in biopharmaceutical products. Pharmaceutical Research, 25(7), 1631-1636. https://doi.org/10.1007/s11095-007-9516-9
7. Arakawa, T., Kita, Y., & Carpenter, J. F. (1991). Protein--solvent interactions in pharmaceutical formulations. Pharmaceutical research, 8(3), 285–291. https://doi.org/10.1023/a:1015825027737
8. U.S. Pharmacopeia (USP). (2021). General Chapter <1150>: Pharmaceutical stability. http://www.uspbpep.com/usp29/v29240/usp29nf24s0_c1150.html
9. Food and Drug Administration (FDA). (2004). Guidance for industry: Analytical procedures and methods validation. https://www.fda.gov/files/drugs/published/Analytical-Procedures-and-Methods-Validation-for-Drugs-and-Biologics.pdf

10. Iyer, H., & Wray, W. (2009). Regulatory aspects of stability testing for biologics. Biopharm International, 22(11), 30-34.
11. Carstensen, J. T., & Rhodes, C. T. (Eds.). (2000). Drug Stability: Principles and Practices. CRC Press.
12. European Medicines Agency (EMA). (2017). Guideline on Process Validation for Finished Products. https://www.ema.europa.eu/en/documents/scientific-guideline/guideline-process-validation-finished-products-information-and-data-be-provided-regulatory-submissions-revision-1_en.pdf
13. Food and Drug Administration (FDA). (2004). Guidance for industry: Changes to an approved NDA or ANDA. https://www.fda.gov/files/drugs/published/Changes-to-an-Approved-NDA-or-ANDA.pdf
14. Food and Drug Administration (FDA). (1999). Revised proposal on site-specific stability data. Retrieved from http://www.triphasepharmasolutions.com/Resources/Stability%20Site%20Changes%20FDA.pdf
15. Coffey, T., & Yang, H. (Eds.). (2018). Statistics for biotechnology process development. CRC Press. https://doi.org/10.1201/9781315120034
16. Chow, S.-C. (2007). Statistical design and analysis of stability studies. Chapman & Hall/CRC Press.
17. International Conference on Harmonisation (ICH). (2002). Bracketing and matrixing designs for stability testing of new drug substances and products (Q1D). https://database.ich.org/sites/default/files/Q1D%20Guideline.pdf
18. International Conference on Harmonisation (ICH). (1995). Quality of biotechnological products: Stability testing of biotechnological/biological products Q5C. Retrieved from https://database.ich.org/sites/default/files/Q5C%20Guideline.pdf
19. International Conference on Harmonisation (ICH). (1999). Specifications: Test procedures and acceptance criteria for biotechnological/biological products Q6B. Retrieved from https://database.ich.org/sites/default/files/Q6B%20Guideline.pdf

20. Chelius, D., Rehder, D. S., & Bondarenko, P. V. (2005). Identification and characterization of deamidation sites in the conserved regions of human immunoglobulin gamma antibodies. Analytical chemistry, 77(18), 6004–6011. https://doi.org/10.1021/ac050672d
21. Wang W. (1999). Instability, stabilization, and formulation of liquid protein pharmaceuticals. International journal of pharmaceutics, 185(2), 129–188. https://doi.org/10.1016/s0378-5173(99)00152-0
22. International Council for Harmonisation of Technical Requirements for Pharmaceuticals for Human Use (ICH). (2022). Q2(R2): Validation of Analytical Procedures. Retrieved from https://database.ich.org/sites/default/files/ICH_Q2-R2_Document_Step2_Guideline_2022_0324.pdf
23. Arakawa, T., Kita, Y., Ejima, D., Tsumoto, K., & Fukada, H. (2006). Aggregation suppression of proteins by arginine during thermal unfolding. Protein and peptide letters, 13(9), 921–927. https://doi.org/10.2174/092986606778256171
24. Chi, E. Y., Krishnan, S., Randolph, T. W., & Carpenter, J. F. (2003). Physical stability of proteins in aqueous solution: mechanism and driving forces in nonnative protein aggregation. Pharmaceutical research, 20(9), 1325–1336. https://doi.org/10.1023/a:1025771421906
25. Stadtman, E. R., & Levine, R. L. (2003). Free radical-mediated oxidation of free amino acids and amino acid residues in proteins. Amino acids, 25(3-4), 207–218. https://doi.org/10.1007/s00726-003-0011-2
26. Winterbourn C. C. (2008). Reconciling the chemistry and biology of reactive oxygen species. Nature Chemical Biology, 4(5), 278–286. https://doi.org/10.1038/nchembio.85
27. Geiger, T., & Clarke, S. (1987). Deamidation, isomerization, and racemization at asparaginyl and aspartyl residues in peptides. Succinimide-linked reactions that contribute to protein degradation. The Journal of Biological Chemistry, 262(2), 785–794. https://pubmed.ncbi.nlm.nih.gov/3805008/
28. Kato, K., Nakayoshi, T., Kurimoto, E., & Oda, A. (2020). Mechanisms of Deamidation of Asparagine Residues and Effects of Main-Chain

Conformation on Activation Energy. International journal of molecular sciences, 21(19), 7035. https://doi.org/10.3390/ijms21197035

29. Shafer, D. E., Inman, J. K., & Lees, A. (2000). Reaction of Tris(2-carboxyethyl) phosphine (TCEP) with maleimide and alpha-haloacyl groups: anomalous elution of TCEP by gel filtration. Analytical biochemistry, 282(1), 161–164. https://doi.org/10.1006/abio.2000.4609
30. Muralidharan, N., Younger, T., Chan, G., Ball, S., Davis, M., & Bolduc, E. (2024). Maintaining protein disulfide-bond stability during culture harvest: Exploring the effects of temperature and oxygen on reduction-reaction kinetics. Bioprocess International, 22(11), E1. November 2024 E-Book. Retrieved from https://www.bioprocessintl.com/product-characterization/ebook-process-related-impurities-from-identification-to-prevention-of-product-variance
31. Liu, H., & May, K. (2012). Disulfide bond structures of IgG molecules: structural variations, chemical modifications and possible impacts to stability and biological function. mAbs, 4(1), 17–23. https://doi.org/10.4161/mabs.4.1.18347
32. Nothaft, H., & Szymanski, C. M. (2010). Protein glycosylation in bacteria: sweeter than ever. Nature reviews. Microbiology, 8(11), 765–778. https://doi.org/10.1038/nrmicro2383
33. Singh, R., Barden, A., Mori, T., & Beilin, L. (2001). Advanced glycation end-products: a review. Diabetologia, 44(2), 129–146. https://doi.org/10.1007/s001250051591
34. International Council for Harmonisation of Technical Requirements for Pharmaceuticals for Human Use (ICH). (2003). ICH harmonised tripartite guideline: Evaluation for stability data (Q1E). https://database.ich.org/sites/default/files/Q1E_Guideline.pdf
35. Thornalley P. J. (2005). Dicarbonyl intermediates in the maillard reaction. Annals of the New York Academy of Sciences, 1043, 111–117. https://doi.org/10.1196/annals.1333.014
36. Houston, P. L. (2001). Chemical kinetics and reaction dynamics. McGraw-Hill.
37. Montgomery, D.C., Peck, E.A., & Vining, G.G. (2021). Introduction to Linear Regression Analysis (6th Edition). Wiley.

38. Tabachnick, B. G., & Fidell, L. S. (2019). Using multivariate statistics (7th ed.). Pearson Education.
39. Food and Drug Administration (FDA). (2004). Guidance for industry: Stability testing of drug substances and drug products.
40. Evers, A., Clénet, D., & Pfeiffer-Marek, S. (2022). Long-Term Stability Prediction for Developability Assessment of Biopharmaceutics Using Advanced Kinetic Modeling. Pharmaceutics, 14(2), 375. https://doi.org/10.3390/pharmaceutics14020375
41. United States Pharmacopeia. (2023). General chapter <1079.2>: Mean kinetic temperature in the evaluation of temperature excursions during storage and transportation of drug products. Retrieved from https://www.uspnf.com/sites/default/files/usp_pdf/EN/USPNF/usp-nf-notices/gc-1079-chapter-prepost-20230127.pdf

Chapter 7: Comprehensive Risk Assessment and Management of Extractables and Leachables in Process Validation for At-Scale Biopharmaceutical Manufacturing.

Abstract

Material risk assessment is a fundamental aspect of biologics manufacturing, directly influencing process validation, regulatory compliance, and patient safety. By systematically identifying and evaluating risks associated with raw materials, manufacturers can address critical factors—including microbial, chemical, and particulate contamination, variability; and product and process impact—that affect product quality and operational efficiency as shown in Figure 1. Aligned with USP <1043> guidance, this manuscript classifies raw materials based on their criticality and examines how various risks can compromise manufacturing outcomes. Through a comprehensive risk scoring system, the assessment process highlights materials with elevated risk profiles, thus enabling the implementation of targeted control measures.

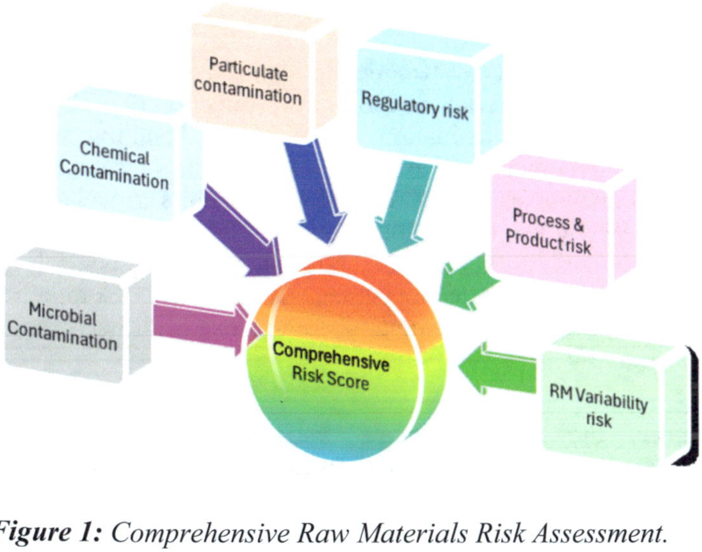

Figure 1: *Comprehensive Raw Materials Risk Assessment.*

Introduction

Raw materials form the foundational elements of safe, high-quality, and efficacious biological products [1-3]. The inherent complexity and sensitivity of biologics necessitate robust risk management strategies [4]. Material risk assessments provide a structured framework to identify and control risks—such as variability, contamination, and instability—that can influence the final product [1,5]. By systematically evaluating raw material criticality, manufacturers maintain compliance with regulatory standards, streamline production processes, and protect patient health [6,7].

This manuscript explores the objectives and significance of material risk assessments, classifies raw materials by their risk profiles, and investigates critical risk categories, including microbial contamination and stability. We present a comprehensive risk scoring system and propose control measures tailored to moderate- and high-risk materials, highlighting the importance of proactive risk management throughout the biologics manufacturing process [1,8].

The Purpose of Material Risk Assessment

Material risk assessments systematically identify, evaluate, and mitigate risks associated with raw materials in biologics production [1]. These assessments address variability, contamination, stability, and handling safety to ensure consistent product quality and efficacy. Raw materials have a direct impact on biological production processes and the final product's critical quality attributes (CQAs) [2,3,9]. By identifying materials with a higher risk of contamination, degradation, or variability, manufacturers can implement controls to safeguard product quality and maintain patient safety [2,9]. Comprehensive risk assessments also facilitate regulatory compliance with agencies such as the FDA, EMA, and ICH [3,10].

Furthermore, they help mitigate variability and microbial or viral contamination risks through appropriate controls [4,11,12]. Thorough assessments enable manufacturers to refine supplier qualification, material handling, and monitoring strategies, ensuring that materials meet required specifications consistently [5,13–15]. This proactive approach reduces disruptions, costs, batch failures, and recalls [6]. Repeated evaluations supply valuable data that support continuous improvement in manufacturing processes, supplier relationships, and overall quality management [7,16]. In summary, material risk assessments are vital for ensuring the safe, effective, and compliant production of biologics [8].

Classification of Raw Material Risks in Biologics Manufacturing

Effective classification of raw materials is essential for maintaining biologics quality, safety, and efficacy. According to USP <1043>, materials are categorized based on their contamination potential, variability, and impurities as summarized in Table 1 and Figure 2 [9,17]. By assigning materials to specific tiers, manufacturers can apply targeted control strategies aligned with each material's risk profile, thereby enhancing the robustness of the manufacturing process.

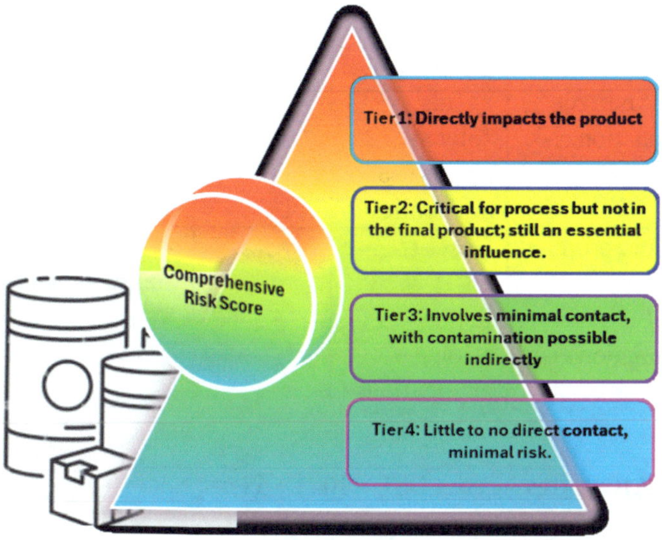

Figure 2: *Tier Classification of Raw Materials Risk per USP<1043>.*

Table 1: Tier Classification of Raw Materials Risk

Tier	Description	Examples	Risk Level	Key Control Strategies
Tier 1	Directly influences product safety, quality, and efficacy high contamination risk	Serum, animal-derived reagents, viral vectors	Highest	Strict sourcing, testing, and regulatory controls [8,9]
Tier 2	Critical but not in the final product; essential for growth/purification	Media supplements, process buffers, critical reagents	Moderate	Consistent quality controls to prevent yield reductions
Tier 3	Minimal product contact; indirect contamination risk via equipment	Cleaning agents, solvents, single-use assemblies	Low	Process controls to prevent particulates/residues
Tier 4	Negligible product interaction; minimal contamination risk	Gases (N_2, CO_2), WFI in non-critical applications	Lowest	Validation for inertness and purity

Common Risk Attributes Across USP <1043> Tiers

Despite tier-based differences, all raw materials share certain key risk attributes, including contamination potential, product and process impact, the need for testing and validation, and supplier reliability [9,17]. Addressing these attributes consistently ensures a robust, compliant production environment that upholds biologics quality.

Contamination Risk (Biological, Chemical, Particulate)

Contamination—biological, chemical, or particulate—can compromise product quality and patient safety [4,11,15,18]. Manufacturers utilize a risk scoring matrix to evaluate contamination risks from 1 (low) to 5 (high), considering sterility, impurity profiles, and handling/storage conditions. Certificates of Analysis (COA) verify compliance with quality specifications [2,3,9].

Biological Contamination

Biological contamination risk is assessed by examining microbial load, endotoxin levels, and viral contaminants, as summarized in Table 2. Materials susceptible to microbial growth demand stricter controls [8,11,12].

Table 2: Biological Contamination Risk Assessment and Scoring

Risk Category (Score)	Description
Low Risk (1)	Minimal microbial growth potential (e.g., inorganic salts, sterile buffers, resins)
Moderate Risk (3)	Some growth potential: sterile but nutrient-rich (e.g., sterile media, WFI, vitamins), Growth-promoting dry nutrient-rich powders where humidity < 1%.
High Risk (5)	Nutrient-rich, prone to contamination (e.g., carbohydrates, animal-derived components)

Chemical Contamination

Material purity, confirmed by COAs and adherence to ICH Q3C and Q3D guidelines, ensures minimal chemical impurities [13–15,19]. Residual solvents, heavy metals, and by-products must be controlled rigorously. Risk scoring guidance for chemical contamination is summarized in Table 3.

Table 3: Chemical Contamination Risk Assessment and Scoring

Category (Score)	Description
Low Risk (1)	High purity (≥98%), no solvents/heavy metals, ICH Q7/Q3C/Q3D compliant [13–15]
Moderate Risk (3)	Some impurities, ≥95% purity, routine testing [14–16]
High Risk (5)	Significant impurities, ≥90% purity, stringent controls and DMF verification [13]

Particulate Contamination

Particulate risk scoring and control involve sterile filtration (0.2 µm), ISO Class 5 cleanrooms, and USP <788> compliance [18–20], as summarized in Table 4.

Table 4: Particulate Contamination Risk Assessment and Scoring

Risk Category (Score)	Description with COA Verification
Low Risk (1)	Stringent particulate control, sterile filtration, ISO Class 5 environment [18–20]
Moderate Risk (3)	Some filtration but not sterile, USP <788> compliance, controlled conditions
High Risk (5)	Minimal particulate control, high particulate levels, inadequate filtration

Product and Process Risk (PPR)

Raw materials can influence CQAs (safety, potency, stability) and overall process performance [1,21]. Directly incorporated materials pose higher risks, while indirect materials can still affect yield, equipment performance, and process reproducibility [22–21]. PPR scoring guidance is summarized in Table 5.

Table 5: Product and Process Risk Assessment and Scoring

Risk Factor	Low Risk (1)	Moderate Risk (2)	High Risk (3)
Product Quality (CQAs)	Minimal CQA impact	Moderate effect on stability, minor interactions	Directly incorporated (e.g., excipient) critical CQAs [21,22]
Process Performance	No effect on consistency/equipment	Some variability, minor equipment impact	High variability, equipment issues, critical step

Regulatory Compliance Risk (RCR)

Compliance ensures that raw materials meet standards set by agencies and compendia. DMF-supported and compendial-grade materials lower regulatory risks. Materials lacking these supports heighten the compliance burden [3,9,22,23,24]. The risk scoring for RCR is summarized in Table 6.

Table 6: Regulatory and Compliance Risk Assessment and Scoring

Risk Category (Score)	Description with COA Verification
Low Risk (1)	DMF-supported or compendial-grade ancillary materials/excipients [9,22,23]
Moderate Risk (3)	Ancillary materials without DMF or compendial status
High Risk (5)	Excipients lacking compendial status [3,24]

Variability Control Risk (VCR)

Material complexity, compendial status, animal origin, and documentation (COA, DMF) affect variability [5,13,14,21]. Simpler, well-characterized materials with robust documentation exhibit lower variability risks.]. The risk scoring for VCR is summarized in Table 6.

Table 7: Variability Control Risk Assessment and Scoring

Risk Category (Score)	Description with COA Verification
Low Risk (1)	Simple, compendial materials with complete COA/DMF documentation
Moderate Risk (3)	Moderately complex, non-compendial, but widely accepted materials
High Risk (5)	Highly complex, non-compendial, no COA/DMF, animal-derived

Comprehensive Overall Risk Score Calculation

A weighted scoring system integrates four key factors: Contamination Risk (30%), Product/Process Impact (30%), Testing/Validation/Variability Control (25%), and Regulatory Compliance (20%) [1,2,21]. Each factor is scored from 1 to 3, and the weighted scores yield a final Weighted Risk Score (WRS) as shown in Equation 1.

Equation (1):

$$WRS_{Total} = (w_1 \times RS_1) + (w_2 \times RS_2) + \cdots + (w_n \times RS_n) \quad \text{Eq (25)}$$

Table 9: Weight Assignment for Risk Categories

Factor	Weight (%)	Explanation
Contamination Risk (CCR)	30%	Direct impact on safety and product integrity [8,9]
Product & Process Impact (PPR)	30%	Ensures product quality and manufacturing efficiency [21]
Testing, Validation, Variability (TVVC)	25%	Ensures consistency, reduces variability [13–16,21]
Regulatory Compliance Risk (RCR)	20%	Ensures alignment with global standards [3,23,24]

Threshold Scores:

- Low Risk (Tier 3/4): ≤ 1.9
- Moderate Risk (Tier 2): 2.0–2.5
- High Risk (Tier 1): 2.6–3.0

Controls in Place for Moderate and High-Risk Materials

After calculating the comprehensive risk score, manufacturers apply appropriate control measures that address the dominant risk factors—whether microbial, chemical, particulate, regulatory, product and process or variability-related. For materials categorized as Tier 2, this often involves enhanced monitoring protocols and minor process adjustments. In contrast, Tier 1 materials demand more stringent interventions, including complete containment, continuous real-time monitoring, and thorough testing, as detailed in Table 8 [1,5]. Meanwhile, for risks classified as Tier 3 and Tier 4, standard monitoring and controls remain adequate, requiring no significant modifications to current procedures.

Table 8: Controls for Moderate and High-Risk Materials

Contamination Type	Tier-2 Risk Controls	Tier-1-Controls
Biological	Sterile filtration, ISO Class 5, viral clearance [8,11,12]	Pathogen-free certification, robust DMF data [23]
Chemical	In-process chromatography, UF/DF washes [13–16]	Enhanced impurity profiling, real-time quality monitoring
Particulate	Filtration (0.2 μm), ISO Class 5 monitoring [18–20]	Intensive particulate control, rigorous USP <788> testing
Product & Process	Real-time CQA monitoring, DMF support [21–21]	Intensive validation, possible process redesign [22–21]

Regulatory Compliance	Standard documentation, validation [3,23,24]	Detailed submissions justifying non-DMF status [3,23,24]
Variability Risk	Increased testing, supplier communication [5,7]	Tightened specifications, dual-sourcing, advanced characterization

Conclusion

Material risk assessments are integral to biologics manufacturing, enabling proactive identification and mitigation of critical risks. By addressing contamination, variability, product and process impacts, and regulatory compliance, manufacturers maintain stable product quality and ensure patient safety [1,7,8]. The comprehensive risk scoring system, coupled with tailored control measures, supports continuous improvement and forms a robust foundation for high-quality biologics production [4–6,9].

References

1. International Conference on Harmonisation (ICH). (2005). *ICH Q9: Quality Risk Management.* Geneva, Switzerland. https://www.ema.europa.eu/en/documents/scientific-guideline/international-conference-harmonisation-technical-requirements-registration-pharmaceuticals-human-use-ich-guideline-q9-r1-quality-risk-management-step-5-revision-1_en.pdf
2. International Conference on Harmonisation (ICH). (2000). *ICH Q7: Good Manufacturing Practice Guide for Active Pharmaceutical Ingredients.* Geneva, Switzerland. https://database.ich.org/sites/default/files/Q7%20Guideline.pdf
3. U.S. Food and Drug Administration (FDA). (2011). *Guidance for Industry: Process Validation: General Principles and Practices.* Silver Spring, MD: FDA. https://www.fda.gov/files/drugs/published/Process-Validation--General-Principles-and-Practices.pdf
4. European Medicines Agency (EMA). (2018). *Guideline on the quality of biologically active substances produced by stable cell lines.* EMA/CHMP/BWP. https://www.tga.gov.au/sites/default/files/2024-07/guidelineonqualityofbiologicalactivesubstancesproducedbytransgeneexpressioninanimalscurrent.pdf
5. World Health Organization (WHO). (2013). *WHO guidelines on good manufacturing practices for biological products.* WHO Technical Report Series. https://www.who.int/docs/default-source/biologicals/gmp/annex-2-who-good-manufacturing-practices-for-biological-products.pdf
6. Rathore, A. S., & Winkle, H. (2009). Quality by design for biopharmaceuticals: Perspectives and challenges. *Nature Biotechnology, 27*(1), 26–34. https://doi.org/10.1038/nbt0109-26
7. International Society for Pharmaceutical Engineering (ISPE). (2011). *ISPE Baseline Guide: Biopharmaceutical Manufacturing Facilities.* ISPE. https://ispe.org/publications/guidance-documents/baseline-guide-vol-6-biopharmaceutical-manufacturing-facilities-3rd-edition
8. International Conference on Harmonisation (ICH). (1999). *ICH Q5A(R1): Viral Safety Evaluation of Biotechnology Products Derived from Cell Lines of Human or Animal Origin.* Geneva, Switzerland. https://database.ich.org/sites/default/files/Q5A%28R1%29%20Guideline_0.pdf

9. United States Pharmacopeial Convention (USP). (2020). *USP General Chapter <1043> Ancillary Materials for Cell, Gene, and Tissue-Engineered Products.*
10. European Pharmacopoeia (Ph. Eur.). (2021). *General chapters on biological products.* Strasbourg, France: EDQM.
11. U.S. Food and Drug Administration (FDA). (2004). *Guidance for Industry: Sterile Drug Products Produced by Aseptic Processing - Current Good Manufacturing Practice.* Silver Spring, MD: FDA. https://www.fda.gov/regulatory-information/search-fda-guidance-documents/sterile-drug-products-produced-aseptic-processing-current-good-manufacturing-practice
12. United States Pharmacopeial Convention (USP). (2020). *USP General Chapter <85> Bacterial Endotoxins Test. https://www.usp.org/harmonization-standards/pdg/general-methods/bacterial-endotoxins*
13. International Conference on Harmonisation (ICH). (2021). *ICH Q3C(R8): Guideline for Residual Solvents.* Geneva, Switzerland. https://database.ich.org/sites/default/files/ICH_Q3C-R8_Guideline_Step4_2021_0422_1.pdf
14. International Conference on Harmonisation (ICH). (2014). *ICH Q3D(R2): Guideline for Elemental Impurities.* Geneva, Switzerland. https://database.ich.org/sites/default/files/Q3D-R2_Guideline_Step4_2022_0308.pdf
15. U.S. Food and Drug Administration (FDA). (2000). *Guidance for Industry: ANDAs: Impurities in Drug Substances.* Silver Spring, MD: FDA. https://www.fda.gov/media/183885/download
16. U.S. Food and Drug Administration (FDA). (2015). *Container Closure Systems for Packaging Human Drugs and Biologics.* Silver Spring, MD: FDA. https://www.fda.gov/media/70788/download
17. United States Pharmacopeial Convention (USP). (2020). *USP General Chapter <788> Particulate Matter in Injections. https://www.uspnf.com/sites/default/files/usp_pdf/EN/USPNF/revisionGeneralChapter788.pdf*
18. European Pharmacopoeia (Ph. Eur.). (2021). *Chapter 2.9.19: Particulate Contamination: Sub-visible Particles.* Strasbourg, France: EDQM.

19. ISO. (2015). *ISO 14644-1:2015 Cleanrooms and associated controlled environments—Part 1: Classification of air cleanliness by particle concentration.* ISO. https://www.iso.org/standard/53394.html
20. International Conference on Harmonisation (ICH). (2009). *ICH Q8(R2): Pharmaceutical Development.* Geneva, Switzerland. https://database.ich.org/sites/default/files/Q8_R2_Guideline.pdf
21. U.S. Food and Drug Administration (FDA). (2019). *Guidance for Industry: Drug Master Files.* Silver Spring, MD: FDA. https://www.fda.gov/media/131861/download
22. Rathore, A. S. (2009). Roadmap for implementation of Quality by Design (QbD) for biotechnology products. *Trends in Biotechnology, 27*(9), 546–553. https://doi.org/10.1016/j.tibtech.2009.05.006
23. European Medicines Agency (EMA). (2016). *Guideline on the requirements for quality documentation concerning biological investigational medicinal products in clinical trials.* EMA/CHMP/BWP. https://www.ema.europa.eu/en/documents/scientific-guideline/guideline-requirements-quality-documentation-concerning-biological-investigational-medicinal-products-clinical-trials-revision-1_en.pdf
24. U.S. Food and Drug Administration (FDA). (2015). *Regulatory Procedures Manual.* Silver Spring, MD: FDA. https://www.fda.gov/inspections-compliance-enforcement-and-criminal-investigations/compliance-manuals/regulatory-procedures-manual

Chapter 8: Comprehensive Risk Assessment and Management of Extractables and Leachables in Process Validation for At-Scale Biopharmaceutical Manufacturing.

Naveenganesh Muralidharan*, Leya S Rose and Mark Davis

Manufacturing Science and Technology (MSAT), AGC Biologics, Boulder, USA

Email address:

nmural@agcbio.com (Naveenganesh Muralidharan)

*Corresponding author

Introduction

Leachable impurities pose a significant challenge during process validation for at-scale commercial manufacturing. These impurities, originating from manufacturing components, process equipment, and packaging materials, can directly impact patient safety through toxicity or compromise the drug's quality and stability. Extractables are chemical compounds that migrate from materials under exaggerated conditions, while leachables are substances that enter the product during normal manufacturing conditions. Leachables may also interact with the drug product to form new impurities, further underscoring the importance of thorough evaluation during process validation [1, 2].

Single-use systems (SUS) have revolutionized biopharmaceutical manufacturing by offering flexibility and cost efficiency. However, SUS components such as bags, tubing, filters, and connectors can introduce extractables and leachables (E&L) into the manufacturing process. These substances, often originating from polymers, elastomers, and other materials, pose risks to product safety, efficacy, and regulatory compliance during commercial-scale operations [3].

This manuscript focuses on risk assessment methodologies tailored for at-scale commercial manufacturing during process validation. It outlines structured approaches to evaluate E&L risks, rationalize risk scoring for SUS components, and establish safety thresholds based on toxicological and analytical considerations. It emphasizes the importance of conducting extractables testing that reflects real-world process conditions and ensures alignment with vendor-provided data.

Chromatography resin extractables and leachables are excluded from this discussion, as regulatory guidance and small-scale studies with vendor-provided data are widely accepted for their assessment. At-scale studies for chromatography resins are considered unnecessary due to the robustness of these established methodologies. Instead, this article centers on single-use system components, where extensive evaluation and risk mitigation strategies are essential to address E&L risks during process validation for commercial-scale manufacturing.

Safety Thresholds for Leachables

Safety thresholds play a pivotal role in prioritizing leachables in risk assessments. The general threshold is set at 1.5 µg/person/day (0.5 ppb) for substances, requiring case-by-case evaluation for chemicals with positive Ames test results or specific structural alerts such as N-nitroso or benzidine-like compounds. For chemicals lacking structural alerts for carcinogenicity or showing negative results in mutagenicity tests (Ames test), the threshold is 15 µg/person/day (5 ppb). A higher threshold of 45 µg/person/day (15 ppb) applies to chemicals without carcinogenicity alerts, with negative mutagenicity test results, and supported by an appropriate acute toxicity test showing LD50 >1000 mg/kg body weight [4].

By leveraging these thresholds, manufacturers can prioritize risk mitigation efforts, focus analytical testing on high-risk leachables, and ensure compliance with safety and regulatory standards. Conducting extractables testing and verifying that vendor-provided data brackets the intended process conditions are critical to aligning leachable profiles with established thresholds.

Risk Assessment Framework

A robust risk assessment framework evaluates SUS components based on their material type, proximity to the drug product, and exposure conditions. Table 1 summarizes the risk factors and scoring criteria for risk factors.

Table 1: Risk Factors for E&L Risk Assessment.

Risk Factor	Low Risk Score:(1)	Medium Risk Score:(2)	High Risk Score	Reference
Proximity to Drug Substance/Product	Early Process Stage	Mid-Process Stage	Final Product Stage	[6]
Contact Time	<1 Hour	1-24 Hours	>24 Hours	
pH	Neutral (6-8)	Slightly Acidic/Basic (4-6 or 8-10)	Strongly Acidic/Basic (<4 or >10)	
Ethanol-related Solvent	No Ethanol	Low Concentration (< 30%)	High Concentration (>30%)	
Temperature	Room Temperature (20-25°C)	Elevated Temperature (25-50 °C)	High Temperature (>50 °C)	
Contact Material	Low Risk (Glass/Steel)	Medium Risk (Elastomer)	High Risk (Plastic/Polymer)	

Assessing these risks allows manufacturers to prioritize mitigation strategies, including enhanced testing, material substitution, or additional compatibility studies. Ensuring that extractables testing aligns with process-specific solvents, temperatures, and contact durations is essential to predict leachables accurately.

Consolidated Risk Score

A consolidated risk-scoring formula integrates multiple factors, including proximity to the drug product, contact time, temperature, and material compatibility. Each factor receives a weight based on its significance, allowing manufacturers to calculate an overall risk score as shown in Equation 1.

$$R_c = (W_p \times R_p) + (W_t \times R_t) + (W_f \times R_f) + (W_{ph} \times R_{ph}) + (W_e \times R_e) + (W_T \times R_T) + (W_m \times R_m) \quad \text{Equation 1}$$

Where R_p, R_t, R_f, R_{ph}, R_e, R_T and R_m represent the risk scores for proximity, contact time, pH, ethanol-related solvents, temperature, and material type, respectively. The corresponding weights (W_p, W_t, etc.) reflect the importance of each factor.

By setting thresholds, such as $Rc \leq 15$ for low risk, $16 \leq Rc \leq 30$ for medium risk, and $Rc > 30$ for high risk, manufacturers can prioritize components and processes that require additional mitigation measures. Components with high scores may necessitate extensive extractables testing, adjustments in material selection, or process modifications.

Risk weightage guidance for Risk Factors

For instance, bag films, bottles, and carboys constructed from polymers exhibit high-risk profiles due to their large surface areas and direct contact with process fluids. Similarly, tubing and connectors, subjected to dynamic flow and varying process conditions, carry significant risks of leachables. In contrast, molded stoppers, typically made of elastomers, pose moderate risks due to the presence of vulcanization agents. Impellers, composed of mixed materials, require separate studies for each material, particularly when exposed to solvents or agitation. Filters with high surface areas and direct solvent exposure also present high risks and demand stringent extractables testing. A summary of the rationale and recommended weightage for these components is provided in Table 2.

Table 2: Risk Factor weightage for E&L Risk Assessment.

Risk Factor	Weightage	Rationale
Proximity to Drug Product	3	Direct correlation to patient safety.
Contact Time	2	Longer durations increase migration risks.
pH	2	Strongly acidic/basic conditions enhance leachable extraction.

Risk Factor	Weightage	Rationale
Ethanol-related Solvent	1	Higher polarity solvents influence extraction but are less critical.
Temperature	2	Elevated temperatures accelerate leachable migration.
Contact Material	2	Determines potential sources of extractables.

Risk assessment guidance for the Biologics manufacturing process stage

Monoclonal antibody (mAb) production involves a series of unit operations classified by their proximity to the Drug Substance (DS) and Drug Product (DP) stages. Early process steps, such as cell culture and harvesting, have lower risks related to contamination and leachables due to dilution and subsequent purification steps. Mid-process steps, including chromatography and virus filtration, involve higher risks as the mAb is purified and concentrated. Final product stages, such as formulation and aseptic filling, are the most critical, as any leachables or extractables (L&E) directly impact patient safety and require the most stringent risk assessments [5].

Table 3 provides a classification of unit operations in mAb production based on their proximity to DS and DP stages. It also highlights the typical single-use components associated with each step and their implications for L&E risk assessments. By understanding these relationships, manufacturers can implement effective control strategies to mitigate risks, ensuring the production of safe and high-quality mAb products.

Table 3: Risk classification on manufacturing process stage based on Unit operation proximity to drug substance and drug product

Classification and Risk Score	Unit Operation	Description	Typical Single-Use Components
Early Process Steps (1)	**Shake Flask and Bags**	Cell expansion from vial through shale flasks and bag bioreactors	Shake flasks, single-use bags, pipettes, filter units.

Classification and Risk Score	Unit Operation	Description	Typical Single-Use Components
	Cell Culture	Gradual scale-up of cell density in seed train bioreactors to large production bioreactors.	Single-use bioreactors, media storage bags, tubing sets, sensors.
	Harvesting	Separation of cells and debris from culture medium using centrifugation or depth filtration.	Depth filters, single-use centrifuge bags, harvest bags, and connectors.
	Clarification	Further removal of insoluble material via filtration.	Depth filtration cartridges, pre-filters, sterile connectors.
Mid-Process Steps (2)	**Protein Capture**	Affinity chromatography (e.g., Protein A/G) for high-purity mAb recovery.	Pre-packed chromatography columns, single-use resin cartridges, and tubing assemblies.
	Intermediate Purification	Removal of impurities using ion exchange (IEX), hydrophobic interaction (HIC), or multimodal chromatography.	Pre-packed IEX/HIC columns, single-use flow paths, and filters.
	Virus Removal/Inactivation	Low-pH holds and virus filtration for viral clearance.	Single-use pH probes, virus filters, and sterile bags for hold steps.
	Polishing	The final purification step is to remove aggregates, host cell proteins, and other trace impurities.	Polishing filters, single-use polishing chromatography columns.
Final Product Stages (2)	**Buffer Exchange and Concentration**	Ultrafiltration/diafiltration (UF/DF) for buffer exchange, concentration, and removal of small molecules.	Single-use TFF cassettes, storage bags, and tubing sets.
	Formulation	Adjustment of the mAb solution into the final buffer for stability and efficacy.	Single-use formulation bags, mixing systems, sterile connectors.

Classification and Risk Score	Unit Operation	Description	Typical Single-Use Components
	Aseptic Filling	Filling of the mAb into vials, syringes, or other containers under sterile conditions.	Single-use filling needles, disposable filling manifolds, sterile tubing.
	Lyophilization (if required)	Freeze-drying the product to enhance stability during storage.	Lyophilization trays single-use storage containers (if needed).

Risk Assessment Guidance for contact material

Components with high surface areas, direct fluid contact, or exposure to solvents (e.g., bag films, tubing, and sterilizing filters) generally carry a high-risk level due to their potential to introduce leachables. Materials like elastomers and metals, often used in molded stoppers or filling needles, are rated with a medium-risk level due to their limited surface area or indirect exposure. This categorization aids in prioritizing components for leachable and extractable testing to ensure product integrity and regulatory compliance. Table 4 summarizes typical single use systems often used in biological manufacturing with risk level and score [3].

Table 4: Risk score for typical single-use materials used in biological manufacturing

Component	Material Type	Risk Level	Score	Rationale
Bag film, bottles, and carboys	Plastic/Polymer	High	3	High surface area with direct contact, prone to leachables under process conditions.
Tubing	Plastic/Polymer	High	3	Extended surface area and dynamic

Component	Material Type	Risk Level	Score	Rationale
				flow increase leachable risks.
Bag ports	Plastic/Polymer	High	3	Direct contact under varying process conditions.
Molded stoppers	Elastomer	Medium	2	Vulcanization agents pose moderate leachable risks.
Impellers	Mixed Materials	Medium	2	Agitation and solvent exposure require separate studies for material components.
TFF cassettes	Polymer Membrane	High	3	High-pressure, high-surface-area membranes in contact with process fluids.
Tubing connectors and disconnectors	Plastic/Polymer	High	3	Direct fluid contact during dynamic flow processes.
Fittings, overmolded junctions	Plastic/Polymer	High	3	Direct solvent interaction under process stress.
Aseptic connectors or disconnectors	Plastic/Polymer	High	3	Direct contact with the final stages

Component	Material Type	Risk Level	Score	Rationale
				increases patient risk.
Sterilizing-grade and process filters	Polymer Membrane	High	3	High surface area and solvent exposure.
Filling needles	Metal	Medium	2	Low leachable risk but used in final stages, requiring evaluation.
Chromatography column housing	Plastic/Polymer	Medium	2	Limited solvent exposure compared to filters.
Small parts (e.g., sensors, O-rings, gaskets)	Elastomer/Metal	Medium	2	Localized leachable risk depends on material composition.

Risk Mitigation Framework for Extractables and Leachables

A structured approach to risk mitigation for extractables and leachables (E&L) begins with evaluating each component against a predefined key criterion. This criterion represents the foundational requirement for ensuring safety and compliance. Meeting the key criterion minimizes the need for further testing or adjustments. However, if the criterion is not satisfied, additional mitigation strategies may be implemented to address potential risks effectively. For medium and high-risk levels, one to two targeted mitigation strategies are typically recommended, as summarized in Table 5.

Table 5: E & L Risk Mitigation Strategies

Key Criterion (1st Level Assessment)	Mitigation Strategies (If Key Criterion is Not Met)
Vendor-supplied extractables data brackets all leachable process conditions.	Replace high-risk materials with low-risk alternatives.
	Clearance Steps in Downstream Processes: Operations such as diafiltration, chromatography washes, or other purification steps can eliminate or dilute potentially extractable residues (PERLs). If these processes effectively remove extractables, the risk level can be reduced by one tier. For example, a "high-risk" component may be downgraded to an "intermediate risk" component.
	Flush or Rinse Steps: Components that undergo flushing or rinsing as part of the manufacturing process can see a significant reduction in extractables. If the waste from flushing does not enter the main process stream, the number and quantity of extractables in the final product are further minimized. This can reduce the component's material reactivity risk by one level.
	Process Dilution: Dilution during manufacturing can mitigate the concentration and impact of extractables. This approach can also reduce the risk level by one-tier.
	Work with vendor-to generate extractables data with representative process condition.

Regulatory Expectations

Regulatory agencies emphasize a risk-based approach to extractables and leachables (E&L) evaluations. The U.S. Food and Drug Administration (FDA) outlines in its guidance on container closure systems for packaging human drugs and biologics that the extent of chemical testing should be determined by a risk assessment of the material's interaction with the drug product [7]. Similarly, the European Medicines Agency (EMA) guides plastic immediate packaging materials, stating that the need for leachables studies should be based on the material's characteristics and its interaction with the medicinal product [8]. Additionally, the International Council for Harmonisation (ICH) reinforces this approach in its Q3E concept paper, which emphasizes that the assessment and control of extractables and leachables should be driven by a science- and risk-based framework [9]. These guidelines collectively support the premise that comprehensive extractables data bracketing all relevant process conditions may be sufficient for low-risk scenarios, whereas for components that have direct and prolonged contact with the drug product, especially under conditions that may promote leaching, product-specific leachables studies are essential to ensure patient safety and product quality.

Conclusion

Proactive management of leachables is essential in biopharmaceutical manufacturing to maintain product quality and patient safety. Manufacturers must align extractables testing with their specific processes, leverage analytical tools effectively, and comply with evolving regulatory expectations. Collaboration with suppliers, combined with robust risk assessments and adherence to industry standards, enables manufacturers to mitigate leachable risks, ensuring both compliance and product reliability.

References

1. United States Pharmacopeia. (2015). USP <1663> Assessment of extractables associated with pharmaceutical packaging/delivery systems. In USP 38–NF 33. Rockville, MD: United States Pharmacopeial Convention. https://www.drugfuture.com/Pharmacopoeia/usp38/data/v38332/usp38nf33s2_c1663.html#usp38nf33s2_c1663
2. United States Pharmacopeia. (2015). USP <1664> Assessment of drug product leachables associated with pharmaceutical packaging/delivery systems. In USP 38–NF 33. Rockville, MD: United States Pharmacopeial Convention.https://www.drugfuture.com/Pharmacopoeia/usp38/data/v38332/usp38nf33s2_c1664.html#usp38nf33s2_c1664
3. Biophorum. (2020, April 22). *Disposables: Extractables testing of polymeric single-use components used in biopharmaceutical manufacturing*. Retrieved from https://www.biophorum.com/download/extractables-testing-of-polymeric-single-use-components-used-in-biopharmaceutical-manufacturing/
4. European Commission Scientific Committee on Consumer Safety (SCCS). (2012). Draft opinion on use of the threshold of toxicological concern (TTC) approach for the safety assessment of chemical substances. European Commission. https://ec.europa.eu/health/ph_risk/committees/documents/sc_o_001.pdf
5. Kelley B. (2009). Industrialization of mAb production technology: the bioprocessing industry at a crossroads. mAbs, 1(5), 443–452. https://doi.org/10.4161/mabs.1.5.9448
6. Mavuleti, R. R., & Pa, K. V. (2024, June 6). Application of the risk evaluation matrix as per USP <665> and <1665> for evaluation of leachables risk from single-use components used in biomanufacturing. BioPharm International. Retrieved from https://www.biopharminternational.com/view/application-of-the-risk-evaluation-matrix-as-per-usp-665-and-1665-for-evaluation-of-leachables-risk-from-single-use-components-used-in-biomanufacturing

7. FDA Guidance: U.S. Food and Drug Administration. (2023). Container closure systems for packaging human drugs and biologics. Retrieved from https://www.fda.gov/media/177449/download
8. EMA Guideline: European Medicines Agency. (2005). Guideline on plastic immediate packaging materials. Retrieved from https://www.ema.europa.eu/en/documents/scientific-guideline/guideline-plastic-immediate-packaging-materials_en.pdf
9. ICH Q3E Concept Paper: International Council for Harmonisation. (2020). ICH Q3E Concept Paper: Assessment and control of extractables and leachables for pharmaceuticals and biologics. Retrieved from https://database.ich.org/sites/default/files/ICH_Q3E_ConceptPaper_2020_0710.pdf

Chapter 9: Continued Process Verification Monitoring: Optimizing Control Chart Design by Reducing the False Alarm Rate and Nuisance Signals

Naveenganesh Muralidharan*, Thatsinee Johnson, Mark Davis

Manufacturing Science and Technology, AGC Biologics, Boulder, USA

Email address:
nmural@agcbio.com (Naveenganesh Muralidharan)
*Corresponding author

Abstract: The Food and Drug Administration's 2011 Process Validation Guidance and International Council for Harmonization Quality Guidelines recommend continued process verification (CPV) as a mandatory requirement for pharmaceutical, biopharmaceutical, and other regulated industries. As a part of product life cycle management, during follow-up through process characterization in stage 1 and process qualification and validation in stage 2, CPV is performed as stage-3 validation during commercial manufacturing to ensure that the process continues to remain within a validated state. CPV requires the collection and analysis of data related to critical quality attributes, critical material attributes, and critical process parameters on a minimum basis to elucidate process control regarding the capability to meet predefined specifications and stability via statistical process control tools. In statistical process control, control charts and Nelson rules are commonly used throughout the industry as statistical tools to monitor and trend data to ensure that a process remains in control. In the control chart, the mean value is taken as the center line, and 3σ limits are placed on either side of the center line. Here, manufactured lots are summarized, trended, and discussed at a cross-functional level at pre-defined intervals (either weekly, bi-weekly or even monthly) based on the batch run rate. A cross-functional team assesses details regarding 1) violation frequency, 2) statistical strength of the signal, 3) violation magnitude and its impact on process or quality, and 4) any potential root causes for out-of-expectation or out-of-trend signals. The cross-functional team must analyze whether any signal identified by the control chart is reliable, rather than a false signal or nuisance signal, and must determine whether corrective action should be taken and justify their decision in the CPV meeting minutes, which are input into the quality-control document system. However, basic control charts are susceptible to false alarms and nuisance alarms. Therefore, it is imperative to understand the assumptions behind control charts and the inherent false alarm rates for different Nelson rules. Hence, in this article, we have detailed the assumptions behind the usage of control charts, the rate of false alarms for different Nelson rules, the impact of skewness and kurtosis of data distribution on the false alarm rate, and methods for optimizing control chart design by reducing false alarm rates and nuisance signals.

Keywords: CPV, Control chart false alarm rate, Control chart skewness and kurtosis, Control chart nuisance signal

1. Introduction

The Food and Drug Administration's (FDA)'s 2011 Process Validation Guidance recommends continued process verification (CPV) during stage-3 process monitoring for drug manufacturers. In CPV, Shewhart control charts are employed as a statistical tool for monitoring process parameters and attributes (critical process parameters (CPPs), Key process parameters (KPPs), In-process controls (IPCs), and release specifications). In control charts, the calculated process average is utilized as the center line, and control limits are placed at $k = \pm 3$ short-term standard deviations (σ_R) away from the process average. The control chart, along with Nelson rules, serves as a tool for detecting out-of-control (OOC) data, defined as data that falls beyond the set control limits, and out-of-trend (OOT) data, defined as a group of data that forms a non-random pattern (shift in mean or increasing/decreasing pattern) [1-3]. Although control charts are commonly applied across the industry to assess the statistical stability of a process, this approach introduces two types of risk: 1) false alarms, i.e., signals that are incorrectly identified as OOC or OOT when the data are actually due to the normal inherent variability of the process itself, and 2) nuisance alarms, i.e., signals that are too small to have any impact on the process or lack sufficient statistical reliability [4, 5]. In practice, small process variations and shifts are anticipated in many processes; therefore, control charts should detect moderate to large shifts that have more practical application rather than small or practically insignificant shift signals. Both high false alarm rates (FARs) and frequent nuisance alarms will reduce the reliability of control chart signals. Therefore, in this article, we provide a review of the current state of understanding on false rate signals arising from the application of Nelson rules, attributes of data distributions and their impact on FARs in the usage of control charts, and methods for reducing FARs by optimizing the usage of Nelson rules and adjusting the value of k (the number of standard deviations from the mean) to accommodate variability and asymmetricity in data distributions.

2. Functional Modules of CPV.

CPV SOP: Drug manufacturers define a standard operating procedure for CPV as a guidance document that minimum should discuss 1) criteria for selection parameters to be monitored and trended, 2) the Frequency of cross-functional team data review meetings to review the trends of parameters and attributes, 3) Participants in the cross-functional CPV data review meeting, 4) Discuss different statistical methods to assess the process capability and stability based on type of data distribution, 5) Method of controlled way of documenting the meeting minutes of CPV data review meeting, 6) Guidance on frequency of CPV report generation based on batch run rate, and 7) Guidance on reaction and response to signals from CPV data monitoring system.

CPV Plan: As per the recommendations in CPV SOP, the CPV plan is generation for each drug substance intermediate stage, which lists out all the parameters to be monitored and trended, type of data distribution and statistical method that may be applied to assess the stability and capability.

CPV data review meeting: As recommended in the CPV SOP, the parameters listed in CPV plans are charted and analyzed for signals of unexpected variation from historical performance as a cross-functional team that includes minimum participation from manufacturing, quality assurance (QA), manufacturing science and technology (MSAT) and quality control (QC). During the data review, the identified statistical process control signals for OOT or OOC are discussed in 1. Magnitude of signal, 2. Statistical reliability of signal 3. Risk of severity on product quality or/and process performance and decision on how to respond to the signal is warranted. If the signal is identified as a nascence signal or not practically significant enough or not statistically significant enough, then no response or action is required. If the signal is identified to be real and has both practical and statistical strength but still not significant enough to impact product quality, then a technical evaluation may be warranted to understand the cause of variation; details of evaluation and results should be followed up in subsequent CPV meetings. If the signal is identified to be real and has both practical statistical significance and magnitude significant enough to impact the product quality potentially, then an investigation under a quality management system may be required.

CPV reports: CPV reports are generated either annually, semiannually or quarterly basis based on batch run rate. Here all parameters and attributes listed in CPV pans are monitored and trended along with summary stability and capability discussions along with all the CPV data review meeting minutes. Recommendations from the CPV reports on changes in the frequency of monitoring or retiring parameters from CPV monitoring may be implemented in CPV plans.

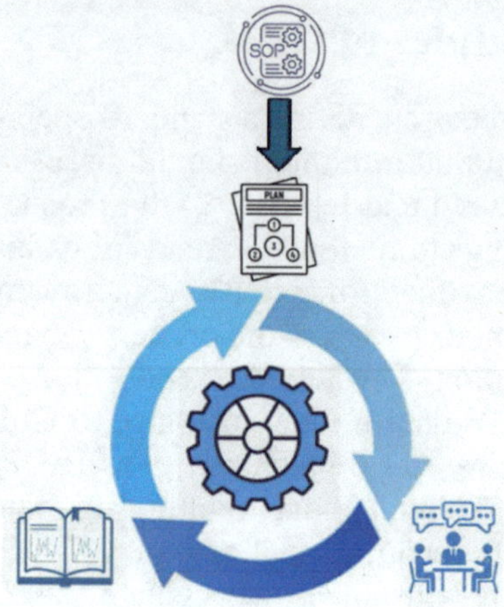

Figure 1. *Functional modules of CPV*

2. FARs in control charts

In 1924, Walter Andrew Shewhart introduced the concept of data analysis using control charts, which was later adopted by the pharmaceutical and biopharmaceutical industries when regulatory agencies requested that drug manufacturers perform CPV [6]. In control charts or XBar charts, the center line is placed at the average, and control limits are typically placed at k standard deviations from the average. Typically, k = 3 is utilized, for which there is a 0.135% probability that any data point belonging to a normally distributed population will fall outside ±3 standard deviations (σ). This approach gives an interval of expected future observations if the process does not change. If observations are within these limits, it can be assumed that the validated state is maintained; if observations are outside these limits, the mean and/or standard deviation has probably changed, potentially requiring attention. σ is often calculated as a short-term σ_R, which causes the limits to be more sensitive to drift, as shown in Equation (1).

$$CL = \mu \pm 3(\sigma_R) \quad (1)$$

The control chart is divided into six zones based on distance from the center line, as shown in Figure 1. Each zone is one standard deviation (σ_R) wide. The 3-σ_R limits on both sides of the center line show the upper control limit and lower control limit. The 2-σ_R limits indicate the upper and lower warning limits, and the 1-σ_R limits on each side of the center line are the upper and lower one-sigma limits. Control charts, along with Nelson rules 1–8 (summarized in Table 1), are used to monitor process control and performance for stability and capability based on the location of data in different zones, the frequency of occurrence of any patterns, and the distance from the mean [6]. To correctly apply the Nelson test rule signals in a control chart, it is imperative to understand the normal, acceptable probability for a data point to fall within or outside of the control chart zones. For instance, for a hypothetical mean μ=0 and standard deviation σ=1, the probability that normally distributed data will fall between -3 SD and +3 SD is given by Equation (2).

$$p = 1 - [\Phi(x = 3) - \Phi(x = 3)] \qquad (2)$$

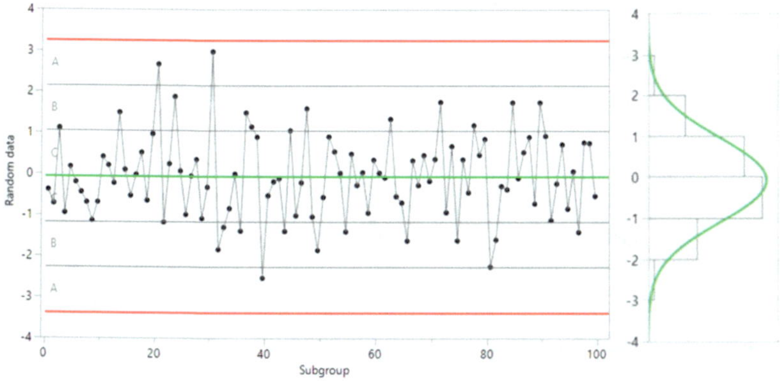

Figure 1. *Sample X control chart constructed from randomly generated data.*

2.1 Optimizing the number of Nelson test rules used in a control chart

In statistical process control, the FAR or rate of type I errors, often identified by the symbol α, indicates the likelihood that data will be falsely identified as an abnormal signal when the data actually correspond to the normal variability of the process. Table 1 summarizes the different Nelson rules and their purposes, along with the probability of a false alarm for each Nelson rule [7]. The FARs from all eight Nelson rules identified in Table 1 sum up to 2.65%. Although it might be intriguing to use all eight Nelson test rules, Nelson (1984) suggested keeping the FAR below 1% [6]. Nelson also stated that tests 5 and 6 should be included only when there is an economic desire to have an early warning, as these rules increase the FAR. Tests 7 and 8 are used to diagnose stratifications and to identify subgroups taken from two different means. Therefore, test rules 7 and 8 have application only when subgroups are used in the control chart. However, in the biopharmaceutical industry, testing is typically performed for a single sample taken from a batch; therefore, unless multiple samples are tested and averaged for the single value reported in the control chart, rules 7 and 8 do not add value for data monitoring and trending. Adhibhatta et al. (2017) showed that Nelson tests 1, 2, and 3 are adequate for monitoring OOC and OOT data, with a combined false alarm probability of 0.94 [8]. Thus, in an effort to limit the FAR to <1.0% and considering the practical application of test rules for biopharmaceuticals, it is recommended that only Nelson test rules 1–3 be utilized in a control chart for biopharmaceutical application.

Table 1. *FARs for different Nelson test rules.*

Test number	Purpose	Probability of false alarm
Rule 1: One data point outside the control limit	Detect OOC data	p fal-Nel(1) = 0.00270
Rule 2: Nine consecutive data points on one side of the center line	Detect a process shift	p fal-Nel(2) = 0.00391
Rule 3: Six consecutive data points either increasing or decreasing	Detect a process drift	p fal-Nel(3) = 0.00278
Rule 4: Fourteen consecutive data points alternating up and down	Detect a process alternating between two states	p fal-Nel(4) = 0.00457
Rule 5: Two out of three data points falling outside two sigmas from the center line	Detect an intermediate shift	p fal-Nel(5) = 0.00306
Rule 6: Four out of five data points falling outside two sigmas from the center line	Detect a small shift	p fal-Nel(6) = 0.00553
Rule 7: Fifteen data points falling within one sigma from the center line	Detect a reduction in process variability	p fal-Nel(7) = 0.00326
Rule 8: Eight consecutive data points falling outside one sigma from the center line	Detect mixed process behavior	p fal-Nel(8) = 0.00010

3. FAR in an OOC signal from a limited sample size

OOC data are detected via Nelson rule 1 when a single data point falls outside 3 SD from the mean, with the assumptions that the data are normally distributed, the underlying true population mean (μ) and population standard deviation (σ) are known, and there is no error due to sampling variability. However, for new products, based on the batch run rate, there is a high likelihood of having a very limited sample size during the first couple of years. For small sample sizes, the estimation of the population mean with the sample mean ($\bar{x}$) and of the population standard deviation with the sample standard deviation (SD) and the establishment of control limits will lead to an increased FAR [9, 14]. The risk of an increased FAR due to limited sample size in control limits has been calculated by Bischak et al. (2007) as a function of the number of standard deviations from the mean (k), the number of samples of observations (n), and the size of the subgroup in each observation (m). As discussed above, biopharmaceutical companies typically perform testing on a single sample taken from a batch; therefore, two subsequent lots are used to calculate the short-term standard deviation, and hence, m is assumed to be 2. The FAR for a limited number of observations or sample size (n) is expressed in Equation (3). Here, C4 is an unbiased estimator of standard deviation. The uncertainty that arises from using the sample standard deviation (SD) instead of the underlying true population standard deviation is compensated for by using an unbiased standard deviation estimator (C4) calculated as a function of subgroup size, as expressed in Equation (4) [10, 13]. Here, Φ is the cumulative normal probability density function.

$$FAR_{(n)} = 2 \times \Phi\left(\frac{-k}{\sqrt{1+\frac{1}{n}\left(1+\frac{k^2(1-C_4^2)}{C_4^2}\right)}}\right) \tag{3}$$

$$C_4 = \left[\frac{\Gamma(\frac{m}{2})}{\Gamma(\frac{m-1}{2})}\right] \times \sqrt{\frac{2}{m-1}} \tag{4}$$

The probability of a false alarm caused by utilizing a limited sample size when setting the control limit at k = 3 (i.e., 3 standard deviations from the mean) is calculated by applying Equations (3) and (4), as shown in Figure 2. Figure 2 shows that the reduction in FAR follows an exponential decay curve; we observe a sharp drop below 5% for a sample size of n = 10, followed by a plateau after approximately n = 30 and a further decrease below 1% at n = 100. Therefore, we recommend using a run chart when the sample size is ≤10, using the calculated control limits as tentative control limits for monitoring and updating control limits for sample sizes of 30–100, and using fixed long-term control limits when the sample size is ≥100. Another alternative solution for mitigating the uncertainty in the calculation of control limits for a small sample size (n < 10) is the use of prediction limits. Prediction limits account for the estimation uncertainty that arises from using the sample standard deviation (SD) by replacing the normal quantile with the t quantile at (n–1) degrees of freedom and also accommodates the uncertainty due to the sample mean by including the standard error of the mean, as expressed in Equation (5).

$$CL = \bar{X} \pm t_{(1-\frac{\alpha}{2},\ n-1)}.SD.\sqrt{1 + 1/n} \qquad (5)$$

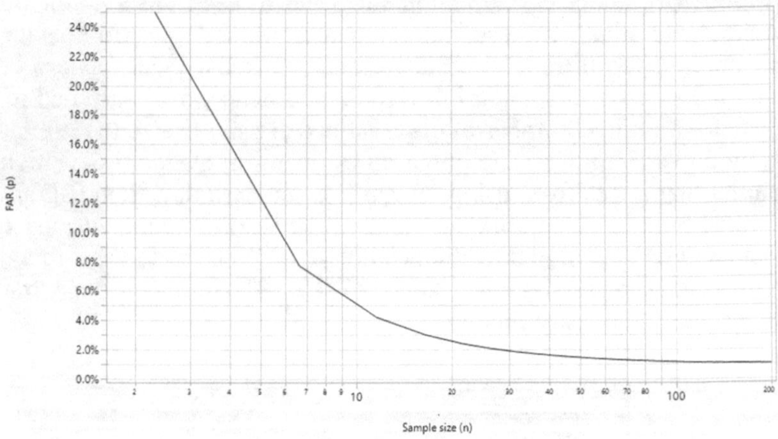

Figure 2. *FAR in an OOC signal from a limited sample size.*

4. FAR in an OOC signal from a skewed or heavy-tailed distribution

The application of Nelson test rules in a control chart is based on a normality assumption. However, if the data are severely skewed or if the variance in the data is excessively broad with a heavy-tailed distribution, this can lead to an increase in the FAR. The asymmetry and tail length in data with reference to a normal distribution are measured as skewness (K3) and kurtosis (K4), respectively [14].

4.1. Modeling FAR for an asymmetric data distribution

Control charts are based on the assumption that data distribution is symmetric on either side of the center average line. However, in practice, the data distribution may be off-centered or asymmetric. Skewness (K_3) is a measure of the degree of asymmetry observed in a data distribution. A distribution can have either right-skewed or left-skewed data or no skew at all. A right-skewed distribution is longer on the right side of its peak, and a left-skewed distribution is longer on the left side of its peak. Skewness in a distribution can be calculated from Equation (6) [11]. A highly skewed distribution can lead to a high FAR in control chart signals. The probability distribution function of a skewed data spread can be modeled by a log-normal distribution [12], which is delineated by two parameters, namely, the shape (Sh) or mean (μ) and the scale parameter (Sc) or standard deviation (σ). The FAR caused by skewness in data distribution with control limits placed at $\pm$ 3 (σ_R) from the mean can be determined by knowing the relationship between the skewness value and shape parameter (Sh). A correlation expression between skewness and shape parameter (Sh) was developed from the data reported by Derya et al. (2012), as shown in Figure 3A [12]. Assuming a scale parameter of Sc = 0 with the shape parameter (Sh) calculated via the correlation shown in Figure 3, the FAR for various degrees of skewness can be calculated via Equation (7), as shown in Figure 3B. Here, k is the number of standard deviations from the mean; for control limits placed at 3 SDs from the mean, k = 3. Figure 3B shows that a skewness below 1.5 keeps the control limit signal at an acceptable FAR of <1.0%.

$$K_3 = \frac{\sum_1^n (X_i - \bar{X})^3}{(n) \times \sigma^3} \qquad (6)$$

$$FAR_{K3} = 1 - \Phi\left(\frac{ln(k) - Sc}{Sh}\right) \qquad (7)$$

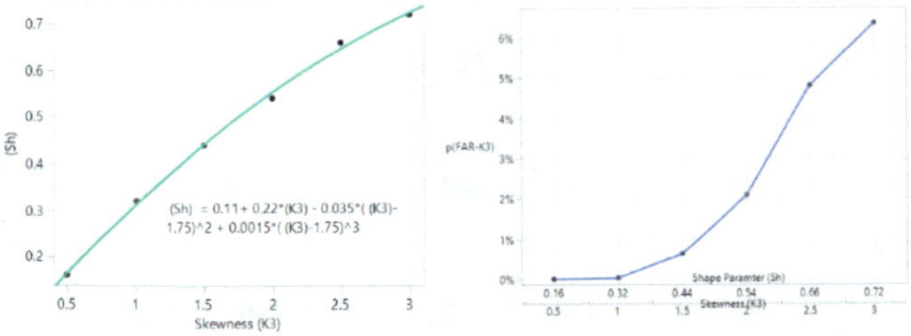

Figure 3. ***(A)*** *Correlation between skewness and log-normal shape factor.* ***(B)*** *FAR for an OOC signal from an asymmetric data distribution.*

4.2. Modeling FAR for a heavy-tailed distribution

Kurtosis is a measure of whether data are heavy-tailed or light-tailed relative to a normal distribution. A data distribution with high kurtosis tends to have heavy tails or outliers. In contrast, a data distribution with low kurtosis tends to have light tails or a lack of outliers. A standard normal distribution has a kurtosis of zero. The kurtosis (K_4) can be calculated from Equation (8) [11, 14]. A positive kurtosis indicates a "heavy-tailed" distribution. A t-distribution has fatter tails than a normal distribution. Therefore, a t-distribution can be used as a model to represent kurtosis, which will allow for a more realistic calculation of the FAR from excess kurtosis [11]. The FAR caused by kurtosis can be modeled via a t-distribution, as expressed in Equation (9) and shown in as shown in Figure 4, by knowing the relationship between kurtosis (K_4) and degrees of freedom (df) for the t-distribution. Here, k is the number of standard deviations from the mean; for control chart limits placed at 3 SDs from the mean, k = 3. df is the number of degrees of freedom for the t-distribution, and $df_{t.\,dist}$ can be calculated from the kurtosis (K_4) in the data distribution, as expressed in Equation (10) [15].

$$K_4 = \frac{\sum_1^n (X_i - \bar{X})^4}{(n) \times \sigma^4} - 3 \qquad (8)$$

$$FAR_{K4} = 2 \times \left[1 - t.dist\big((k), (df_{t.dist})\big)\right] \qquad (9)$$

$$df_{t.dist} = 4 + \left(\frac{6}{K4 - 1}\right) \qquad (10)$$

4.3 Adjustment to k to accommodate skewed and heavy-tailed distributions.

Braden et al. (2022) showed that the FAR for a severely skewed or heavy-tailed distribution can be reduced by replacing the control limits at k = 3 (σ_R) from the mean with limits based on adjusted k values (k'), as expressed in Equations (11) and (12), to accommodate skewness or heavy tails in the data distribution. Branden also stated that Equations (11) and (12) are valid only when the skewness or kurtosis of the distribution meets the criteria expressed in Equation (13) [14]. The factor adjustment for skewness and kurtosis is shown in Figure

(5).

$$k' = 3 + \frac{4}{3}\left(\frac{K_3}{\sqrt{n}}\right) \tag{11}$$

$$k' = 3 + \left(\frac{K_4}{n+0.33\,K_4}\right) \tag{12}$$

$$-2.489 \leq \frac{K_3}{\sqrt{n}} \leq 2.489 \; and \; 0 \leq \frac{K_4}{n} \leq 11.549 \tag{13}$$

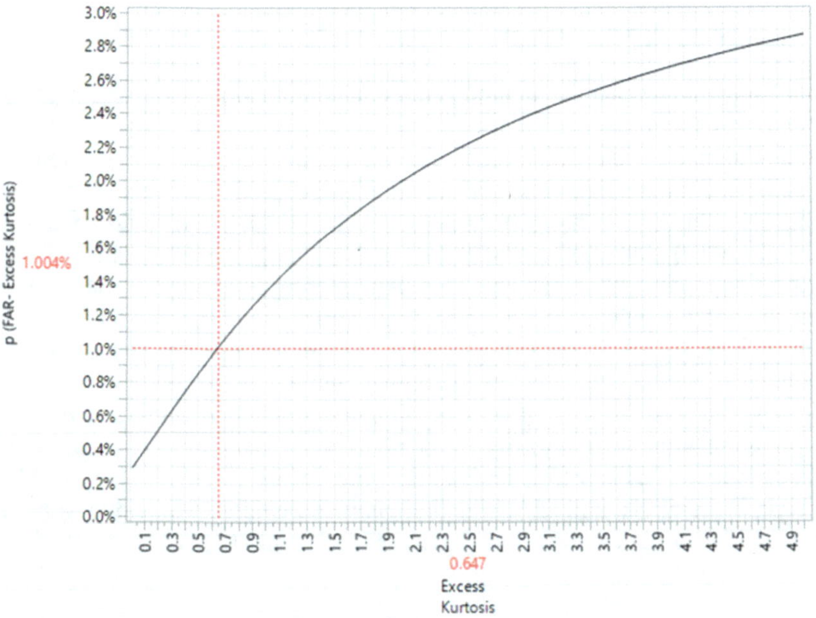

Figure 4. *FAR in an OOC signal due to kurtosis.*

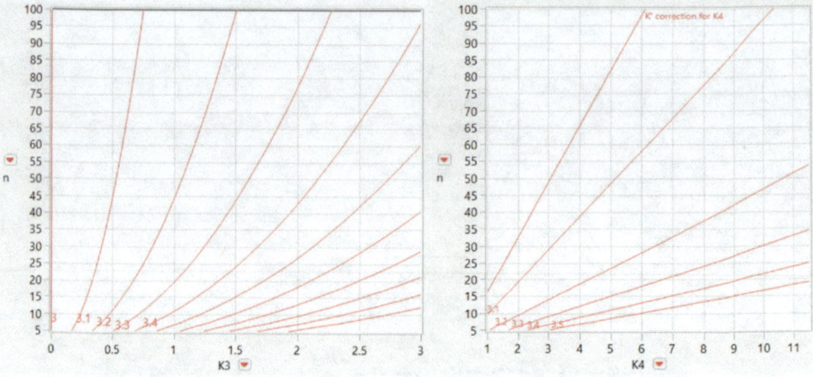

Figure 5. (Left) *Adjustment of k for skewness.* ***(Right).*** *Adjustment of k for kurtosis.*

5. Nuisance signal from Nelson rule 2 and its reliability

According to Nelson rule 2, nine consecutive data points on one side of the center line can be used to detect a shift in the mean, which can result in a nuisance signal, as the magnitude of this shift in the mean can be potentially insignificant. Therefore, when a signal is identified for Nelson rule 2, the strength of the signal must be assessed against the magnitude of the shift. Wheeler (2010) classified a small shift in the mean as a mean shift of <1.5 in terms of the standard deviation (Δ/σ). An intermediate shift is classified as a mean shift of 1.5 ≥ (Δ/σ) ≥ 2.5, and a large shift is classified as a mean shift of (Δ/σ) > 2.5 [16]. The reliability of the signal for the desired shift can be calculated from the type II error. In control charts, the (β) value or type II error indicates the probability of a true signal going undetected. The widely acceptable minimum probability for β is 0.20 [17], which indicates a reliability (1–β) of 100% – 20% = 80%. The relationship between sample size, type I error (α), type II error (β), and (Δ/σ) for the mean is expressed as a two-sided limit and one-sided limit, as shown in Equations (12) and (13) [21].

$$n_T = \frac{\left(t_{1-\alpha/2,df} + t_{1-\beta,df}\right)^2}{\left(\frac{\Delta}{\sigma}\right)^2} \qquad (12)$$

$$n_T = \frac{\left(t_{1-\alpha,df} + t_{1-\beta,df}\right)^2}{\left(\frac{\Delta}{\sigma}\right)^2} \qquad (13)$$

Here, n_T is the total sample size in the analysis, where $n_T = n_{his} + n_{sis}$. n_{his} is the number of historic samples, and n_{Sis} is the number of data points on one side of the center line showing a positive signal for Nelson test rule 2; therefore, n_{Sis} = 2. df = $n_{sig} + n_{his} - 2$, which represents the degrees of freedom, and $t_{(1-\alpha,\ df)}$ represents the inverse of the cumulative t-distribution at 1 – α and df.

Here, an acceptable value of the significance (α) value or type I error is often set at 0.05 [18], indicating a 5% probability of falsely identifying a signal as positive when the data actually correspond to normal variability within the process. In this case, the statistical confidence (1 – α) is 100% – 5% = 95%.

The detectability/shift from the mean (Δ/σ) is the acceptable distance from the mean, expressed as a number of standard deviations. A (Δ/σ) value of 1.0–1.5 has been reported as acceptable for calculating the required sample size [19]. The FDA guidance document on "statistical review and evaluation" states that a (Δ/σ) value of 1.5 at 90% confidence (1 – α) is adequate to conclude equivalence between two groups [20].

Equations (14) and (15) for the sample size are rearranged to solve for the power of estimation, where t.dist is the cumulative distribution function for a one-sided or two-sided t-distribution, respectively. According to Cohen (1988), the generally accepted minimum power (1 – β) is 80% for a confidence (1 – α) of 95% [17]. Figure 6 shows the reliability of a signal for Nelson rule 2 for different combinations of the shift from the mean (Δ/σ) and historic sample size. Assuming a historic data sample size of n_{his} = 30 and a sample size of n_{sis} = 9 on one side of the center line for the Nelson test rule signal, the reliability is calculated via Equation (14) for different values of the shift from the mean (Δ/σ), as shown in Figure 6. Figure 6 demonstrates that if the observed shift in the mean is ≤1 SD, then the signal can be considered as a nuisance signal without sufficient reliability.

$$Power\ (1-\beta) = t.dist\left(\left(\frac{\left(\frac{\Delta}{\sigma}\right)}{\sqrt{\frac{1}{n_{sig}} + \frac{1}{n_{his}}}} - t_{(1-\alpha/2,\ df)}\right), (df)\right) \qquad (14)$$

$$Power\ (1-\beta) = t.dist\left(\left(\frac{\left(\frac{\Delta}{\sigma}\right)}{\sqrt{\frac{1}{n_{sig}}+\frac{1}{n_{his}}}} - t_{(1-\alpha,\ df)}\right), (df)\right) \tag{15}$$

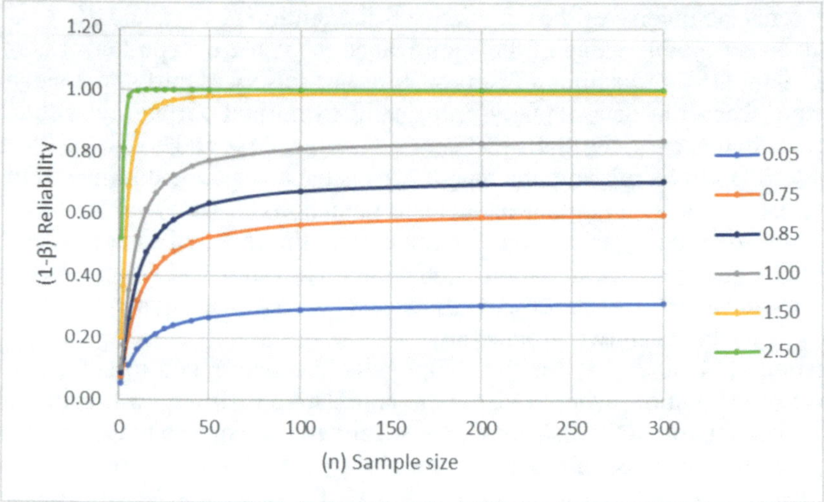

Figure 6. *Reliability vs. sample size for different values of Δ/σ.*

6. Conclusions

Challenges in CPV review sessions include assessing a control chart signal for reliability and deciding whether to initiate an investigation followed by action for corrective or preventive action. However, control charts are susceptible to false alarms and nuisance alarms. Trusting incorrect signals from the control chart and initiating quality control actions can lead to a waste of resources and time. Therefore, it is imperative to understand false alarm probabilities in control charts in association with different Nelson test rules. In this article, we reviewed the current state of understanding of FARs inherent to control charts and the impact on FARs of data distributions that deviate from normal distribution assumptions. We also discussed methods for optimizing the use of control charts by selecting the Nelson test rules to be applied and correcting the number of sigma factors (k) used for calculating control limits to accommodate skewness and kurtosis in a data distribution to reduce the FAR and nuisance signals and to improve the reliability of data trending and monitoring.

Abbreviations

df: Degrees of freedom
FAR: False alarm rate
SD: Standard deviation
OOC: Out-Of-Control
Xbar: Sample mean
p: Probability
nsig = 9: Number samples on one side of the control chart
nhis: Number of samples used for historic samples
K3: Kurtosis
K4: Skewness
k: Number of standard deviations from the mean for the placement of control limits
Δ/σ: Number of standard deviations from the mean for considering the reliability of a shift in the mean
β: Type II error
α: Type I error
μ: Population mean
σ: Population standard deviation
Φ: Cumulative normal density function

References

1. Guidance for Industry: Process Validation — General Principles and Practices. US Food and Drug Administration: Silver Spring, MD, 2011; https://www.fda.gov/files/drugs/published/Process-Validation–General-Principles-and-Practices.pdf.

2. PDA Technical Report 59: Utilization of Statistical Methods for Production Monitoring. Parenteral Drug Association, Bethesda, MD, 2012; https://www.pda.org/bookstore/product-detail/1842-tr-59-utilization-of-statistical-methods.

3. Heigl, N., Schmelzer, B., Innerbichler, F., & Shivhare, M. (2021). Statistical quality and process control in Biopharmaceutical manufacturing—Practical issues and remedies. *PDA Journal of Pharmaceutical Science and Technology*, *75*(5), 425-444. https://doi.org/10.5731/pdajpst.2020.011676

4. Adams, B. M., Woodall, W. H., & Lowry, C. A. (1992). The use (and misuse) of false alarm probabilities in control chart design. Frontiers in Statistical Quality Control 4, 155-168. https://doi.org/10.1007/978-3-662-11789-7_11

5. Walker, E., Philpot, J. W., & Clement, J. (1991). False signal rates for the Shewhart control chart with supplementary runs tests. Journal of Quality Technology, 23(3), 247-252. https://doi.org/10.1080/00224065.1991.11979330

6. Nelson, L. S. (1984). The Shewhart control chart—Tests for special causes. Journal of Quality Technology, 16(4), 237-239. https://doi.org/10.1080/00224065.1984.11978921

7. Griffiths, D., Bunder, M., Gulati, C., & Onizawa, T. (2010). The probability of an out of control signal from Nelson's supplementary zig-zag test. Journal of Statistical Theory and Practice, 4(4), 609-615. https://doi.org/10.1080/15598608.2010.10412007

8. Adhibhatta, S., DiMartino, M., Falcon, R., Haman, E., Legg, K., Payne, R., Pipkins, K., & Zamamiri, A. (2017, February). Continued process verification (CPV) signal responses in Biopharma. ISPE | International Society for Pharmaceutical Engineering. https://ispe.org/pharmaceutical-engineering/january-february-2017/continued-process-verification-cpv-signal

9. Trietsch, D., & Bishak, D. (2007). The Rate of False Signals for Control Charts with Limits Estimated from Small Samples. Journal of Quality Technology, 39(1), 52-63. https://prism.ucalgary.ca/server/api/core/bitstreams/dae8e651-1a93-4337-a3a1-1c2dbe3ae66c/content

10. Bischak, D. P., & Trietsch, D. (2007). The rate of false signals in u control charts with estimated limits. Journal of Quality Technology, 39(1), 54-65. https://doi.org/10.1080/00224065.2007.11917673

11. Richard A. Groeneveld, Glen Meeden, Measuring Skewness and Kurtosis, Journal of the Royal Statistical Society Series D: The Statistician, Volume 33, Issue 4, December 1984, Pages 391–399, https://doi.org/10.2307/2987742

12. Karagöz, D., & Hamurkaroğlu, C. (2012). Control charts for skewed distributions : Weibull, gamma, and lognormal. Metodološki Zvezki, 9(2), 95–106. Repository of the University of Ljubljana. http://www.stat-d.si/mz/mz9.1/karagoz.pdf

13. Munoz, J., Moya Fernandez, P., Alvarez, E., & Blanco-Encomienda, F. (2020). An alternative expression for the constant c4[n] with desirable properties. Scientia Iranica, 0(0), 0-0. https://doi.org/10.24200/sci.2020.52702.2846

14. Braden, P., & Matis, T. (2022). Cornish–fisher-based control charts inclusive of skewness and kurtosis measures for monitoring the mean of a process. Symmetry, 14(6), 1176. https://doi.org/10.3390/sym14061176

15. Kenneth L. Lange, Roderick J. A. Little & Jeremy M. G. Taylor (1989)

Robust Statistical Modeling Using the t Distribution, Journal of the American Statistical Association, 84:408, 881-896, DOI: 10.1080/01621459.1989.10478852

16. Wheeler, D. J., & Chambers, D. S. (2010). Understanding statistical process control. SPC Press.

17. Cohen J. Statistical Power Analysis for the Behavioral Sciences (Second Edition). Lawrence Erlbaum Associates: Hillsdale, NJ, 1988.

18. Kim H. Y. (2015). Statistical notes for clinical researchers: Type I and type II errors in statistical decision. Restorative dentistry & endodontics, 40(3), 249–252. https://doi.org/10.5395/rde.2015.40.3.249

19. Durivage M. How To Establish Sample Sizes for Process Validation Using Statistical Tolerance Intervals. Bioprocess Online 27 October 2016; https://www.bioprocessonline.com/doc/how-to-establish-sample-sizes-for-process-validation-using-statistical-tolerance-intervals-0001.

20. Weng Y. Statistical Review and Evaluation. US Food and Drug Administration: Rockville, MD, 21 March 2016; https://www.fda.gov/media/105013/download.

21. NIST/SEMATECH. Engineering Statistics Handbook. National Institute of Standards and Technology: Gaithersburg, MD, 2012; https://doi.org/10.18434/M32189

Chapter 10: Statistical Methodologies to establish Control or Alert limits for Nonparametric distributed numeric variables with a focus on Bio-Pharmaceutical.

Naveenganesh Muralidharan

Introduction

According to the FDA's 2011 Process Validation Guidance, critical quality attributes and critical process parameters are trended to assess the statistical stability and ability to meet acceptable criteria as a part of a continuous process verification program using control charts. In the control charts, control limits (CL) are used to assess the statistical stability of the process parameters and attributes. When the data are normally distributed, control limits are established in a straightforward manner by placing the control limits three standard deviations away from the process average [1]. However, biological industry data are often not normally distributed, and therefore a regular I-chart with control limits placed three standard deviations from the process mean cannot be used. These data include censored data, which are often reported as being below the limit of quantification (LOQ); trending mutually exclusive events (e.g., fraction of defective items), whose data follow a binomial distribution; or zero-inflated data, which are often reported as zeros that follow a negative binomial distribution. Herein, we describe a detailed step-by-step procedure using Excel formulas for easy establishment of alert limits or statistical control limits for non-normally distributed censored data, binomially distributed data and negative binomially distributed data. For the below discussed statistical alert limit setting methods for non-normally distributed data, it has been shown that a minimum of 25 to 30 samples are required to estimate the mean and standard deviation at acceptable levels of confidence. Furthermore, the data set should have minimum of 4 to 5 discrete values, if not, un-rounded data can be used for the parameter estimation in the below-discussed methods [2].

Censored Data

In bio-pharmaceutical industries, safety-related contaminants, such as endotoxin, or product/process related trace contaminants, are often reported as being below the LOQ, because of the limitations of analytical methods.

Restricted maximum likelihood methods (RML), originally proposed by Persson and Rootzen in 1977, have been suggested to be a more appropriate method for estimating unbiased process averages and standard deviations for censored data [2]. The alert limits can be placed three unbiased standard deviations away from the unbiased process average. This RML method is used, when the number of samples reported as LOQ are up to 50% of the total sample size, if the number of LOQ samples are greater than 50%, it is recommended to trend the data using a run chart or frequency table [2]. The unbiased mean and unbiased standard deviation for censored data can be estimated as shown below [2,3]:

Table 1: Unbiased mean and unbiased standard deviation for censored data
Value below which the results are reported as below the LOQ, X_0
Total number of samples, n
Number of samples reported as below the LOQ, n_{LOQ}
Number samples reported as above the LOQ: $K = n - n_{LOQ}$
λ = NORM.S.INV(n_{LOQ} /n)
Calculate A (only for the samples reported as above the LOQ) = $\Sigma(x_i - x_0)$
Calculate B (only for the samples reported as above the LOQ) = $\Sigma(x_i - x_0)^2$
Calculate biased sigma: $\sigma *= \frac{1}{2}\left(\frac{\lambda . A}{k}\right) + \left[\left(\left(\frac{\lambda . A}{k}\right)^2\right) + 4\left(\frac{B}{k}\right)\right]^{1/2}$
Calculate biased mean: $\mu^* = 1 - (\lambda . \sigma^*)$
Calculate unbiased mean estimators: $B_\mu = -EXP(1)^{\left[2.692 - \frac{(5.439\,(n-k))}{(n+1)}\right]}$
Calculate unbiased sigma estimators: $B_\sigma = -\left[0.312 + \frac{(0.859\,(n-k))}{(n+1)}\right]^2$

Table 1: Unbiased mean and unbiased standard deviation for censored data
Calculate unbiased mean: $$\mu = \mu^* - \left(\frac{\sigma^* . B_\mu}{n+1}\right)$$
Calculate unbiased overall sigma: $$\sigma = \sigma^* - \left(\frac{\sigma^* . B_\sigma}{n+1}\right)$$

Binomially Distributed Data

The proportion or fraction of defective items in a population is often trended in the pharmaceutical industry at the drug product stage. Typically, vials filled with drug products are inspected for one or more quality attributes (e.g., fill volume, particles in the vial filled with solution, proper screwing of vial caps shut or proper labeling of vials) are inspected simultaneously. If only one attribute does not meet the predefined acceptable standard, the item is classified as defective. The fraction or proportion of defective items is often expressed as a percentage for trending the batch performance because the sample size typically differs among batches. Furthermore, the proportion of defective items in successive batches is independent of the previous defective rate; therefore, the probability of the proportion of nonconforming events follows a binomial distribution. The calculation of alert limits for binomially distributed data is a two-step process: first, the confidence interval is calculated with the Clopper-Pearson exact binomial method, and then the tolerance bound at a tolerance interval of 99% is calculated with the method of Hahn and Chandra [4–7].

Step 1: Calculation of the upper confidence bound or confidence interval for the proportion defective in the process
Total sample number, n
Number of defects, x
Calculate the proportion defective in the current process, $p_0 = x/n$
Acceptable risk (default 0.05), α

Step 1: Calculation of the upper confidence bound or confidence interval for the proportion defective in the process
Calculate confidence, $(1-\alpha)$
Calculate upper confidence bound for the estimate of the population mean proportion defective: CL_u= Beta.Inv(1-α,x+1,n-x)
Step 2: Calculation of the upper tolerance bound for the number of defects in an average batch size
Proportion for tolerance interval, (P_r) default value = 0.99
Average sample size per batch, n_A
Upper tolerance bound per n samples per batch: N_u = Binom.Inv (n_A,CL_u,P_r)
Calculation of tolerance bound as a percentage
% Upper tolerance bound, % N_u = 100 x N_u/n

Negative Binomially Distributed Data

Data for environmental monitoring in biopharmaceutical manufacturing clean rooms (e.g., particle counts or bioburden), are often reported as zeros. These data follow a negative binomial distribution, and the data distribution is modeled on the basis of both the chance of occurrence of an event and the intensity of event.

The negative binomial distribution is characterized by two parameters: μ and k, where k is typically termed the negative binomial dispersion parameter, and μ is the mean. Various methods are available for estimating the μ and k. Here in, both parameters are estimated with the simplest method, called method of moments. Furthermore, because a negative binomial distribution is not a symmetric distribution, using a quantile limit is more appropriate than using limits three standard deviations above and below the mean. [8].

Let Xi denote the count of the particles or bioburden, where (i = 1, 2, 3......n)

Calculation of alert limit for negatively distributed data
Calculate the average, μ = Average (X)
Calculate the sample variance, σ^2 = VAR.S (X)

Calculation of alert limit for negatively distributed data
Calculate the dispersion coefficient: $$K = \frac{\sigma^2 - \mu}{\mu^2}$$
Calculate the probability density function (PDF) for each X_i value: $$PDF_{X=i} = ((K * \mu)^\wedge X_i)/(1 + K * \mu)^\wedge(X_i + (1/K)) * ((GAMMA(X_i + (1/K)))/((FACT(X_i)) * GAMMA(1/K)))$$
Calculate the cumulative probability density function (CPDF) at each X_i value: $$CPDF_{X=i} = PDF_i + \sum_{X=0}^{X=i-1} PDF_{X=i}$$
The alert limit can be placed at 0.99 quantile; therefore the alert limit can be identified by placing it at an X value corresponding to $CPDF_{x=i} = 0.99$

References:

1. *Utilization of statistical methods for production monitoring*. (2012). Parenteral Drug Association. https://www.pda.org/bookstore/product-detail/1842-tr-59-utilization-of-statistical-methods
2. Heigl, N., Schmelzer, B., Innerbichler, F., & Shivhare, M. (2021). Statistical Quality and Process Control in Biopharmaceutical Manufacturing-Practical Issues and Remedies. *PDA journal of pharmaceutical science and technology*, *75*(5), 425–444. https://doi.org/10.5731/pdajpst.2020.011676
3. Gibbons, R. D. (1994). Statistical methods for groundwater monitoring. John Wiley & Sons.
4. Hahn, G. J., & Chandra, R. (1981). Tolerance intervals for Poisson and binomial variables. Journal of Quality Technology, 13(2), 100-110. https://doi.org/10.1080/00224065.1981.11980998
5. Agresti, A., & Coull, B. A. (1998). Approximate is better than "Exact" for interval estimation of binomial proportions. The American Statistician, 52(2), 119. https://doi.org/10.2307/2685469
6. Binomial parameter, Clopper-Pearson interval estimation. (2014). Wiley StatsRef: Statistics Reference Online. https://doi.org/10.1002/9781118445112.stat01453
7. Meeker, W. Q., Hahn, G. J., & Escobar, L. A. (2017). Statistical intervals: A guide for practitioners and researchers. John Wiley & Sons.
8. Hoffman, D. (2003). Negative binomial control limits for count data with extra-Poisson variation. Pharmaceutical Statistics, 2(2), 127-132. https://doi.org/10.1002/pst.51

Chapter 11: Process Validation: Pre-Filtration Dirty-Hold Time for Upstream Media and Feed Solutions and its Implications for Establishing In-Process Microbial Control

Naveenganesh Muralidharan, Emma Bolduc, Thatsinee Johnson and Mark Davis

Introduction

Biopharmaceutical manufacturing processes require that prepared raw materials and product intermediates be held at different stages of the process. However, during the hold time, the process and product intermediates are susceptible to microbial risk due to the presence of bioburden, endotoxins, and exotoxins. Microbial risks arise from a variety of sources, including the facility, equipment, process operations, source of raw materials used, and microbial growth-promoting nature of the prepared intermediate material itself.

The Food and Drug Administration's Guidance for Industry Sterile Drug Products Produced by Aseptic Processing states that "the time limits established for the various production phases should be supported by at-scale data. Bioburden and endotoxin load should be assessed when establishing time limits" [1]. Furthermore, United States Pharmacopeial USP<1115> states that "manufacturers must properly establish processing hold times considering whether processing steps and hold times could result in changes to bioburden" [2,3]. Therefore, studies on the pre-sterilization filtration hold time must be performed at the manufacturing scale in order to generate microbial data to ensure that the change in microbial load is controlled before the sterilization process.

Preferably, studies on the pre-sterilization microbial hold time should be performed during engineering runs prior to process performance qualification (PPQ) runs or at least during the PPQ runs. Once the maximum pre-filtration hold times are established before or during the PPQ batches, the routine microbial monitoring for pre-filtration upstream media and feed solutions samples may not be required during regular production batches. However, periodic non-routine sampling and monitoring may be performed annually or after a prolonged shutdown period [11]. Furthermore, the unprocessed bulk harvest [UB] samples taken from the production bioreactor are tested for bioburden and endotoxin from all manufacturing batches. The UB sample from production bioreactor is a representative of the entire upstream processes, including raw materials, media, and feed solutions. Hence, the routine monitoring and sampling of pre-filtration media and feed solutions will be a redundant check and may not be value added to the microbial control strategy of upstream process.

The upstream cell culture media and feed solutions are often sterilized via 0.22-μm filtration. Therefore, pre-sterilization is also referred to as pre-filtration in this article.

Upstream cell culture growth and production media are nutrient-rich, with a neutral pH and a preparation temperature of 25°C – 40°C that supports the growth of most microbes [3]. Therefore, this article emphasizes quantifiable risk assessment methodology for determining the appropriate pre-filtration hold time to ensure that the microbial risk is suitably controlled during the manufacturing process. The risk assessment is based on a conservative calculation that models the change in bioburden load, risk of filtration failure, and impurity safety factor for exotoxins and endotoxins.

Pre-Filtration Hold Time Challenge for Assessment: At our company's facility, among all of the batch volumes prepared in upstream operations, the longest preparation time corresponds to the 20,000-L production bioreactor cell culture media. Although medium preparation and filtration are typically performed within a duration of Tp= 3 hours) from the time of addition of the first component, a four-fold longer preparation time (4Tp) is assessed as a challenge for microbial control. The selection of 4Tp= 12 hours assumes that this four-fold preparation time is a good approximation for addressing any unforeseen issues in manufacturing operations.

Data-based Microbial Load at Time t=0: In-house pre-filtration microbial hold samples at time t=0 have been consistently shown to have a bioburden of ≤ 1 colony-forming units (CFU)/mL for a sample size of 12. However, the cell culture medium preparation is performed in a sanitary, controlled Class-8 clean room rather than a sterile environment. Therefore, there should be some amount of microbial load at the initial time point.

As with any other assay, the bioburden assay is also prone to false-negative results. False negative errors in bioburden analysis might be from non-homogeneous bioburden distribution in test solution, sample handling error from pipetting during dilutions, and recovery efficiency of bioburden in assay. In the above-listed errors, both non-homogeneous bioburden distribution and sampling handling errors are inherent to the method itself. However, error in the recovery of micro-organism in bioburden assay is attributed to bioburden density in the test solution and the test volume that are specific to the process. Low bioburden test volume and low microbial load in test solution can both increase the chances of false negative results. In such instances, when bioburden results of the non-sterile sample are reported as below the detectable limit, then the most probable bioburden concentration in the test solution can be calculated for an acceptable chance false negative results as detailed in step-1 and step-2, as discussed below based on the method detailed by Yang (2013).

False negative error from bioburden test volume and bioburden density in test solution:

The European Medicines Agency (EMA) recommends a minimum of 100 mL as the test volume for a bioburden assay, with 10 CFU as an acceptable limit for the pre-sterile filtration bioburden for sterile drug products. Yang (2013) showed relationship between the false acceptance probability Vs bioburden test volume and bioburden density in test solution. Yang (2013) statistically showed that the sensitivity of a bioburden assay in EMA recommended 100-mL test volume to detect 10 CFU is 41.2%; in other words, the probability of falsely accepting a contaminated batch is (100%–41.2%=58.8%). Now, using this information, Field. R (2013) showed the minimum bioburden level in the test solution for different test volumes below 100mL to have a detectability equivalent to 41.2% [36]. Eq.1 is derived from the data provided by Field R (2013) using non-linear exponential 5-P decay model with JMP14.

Step-1: Using Eq.1, one can calculate what is the minimum bioburden limit in a specific test volume to have an assay sensitivity of 41.2%.

$$CFU/100mL_{41.2\%} = 9.87 + 3.6e^{(-0.033v_t)} + 16.4^{(-0.15v_t)} \qquad \text{Eq. (1)}$$

Here, CFU/100mL41.2% is the minimum bioburden load in test solution at different bioburden test volumes Vt to have a sensitivity of 41.2%, which is equal to detect 10 CFU in 100-mL test volume.

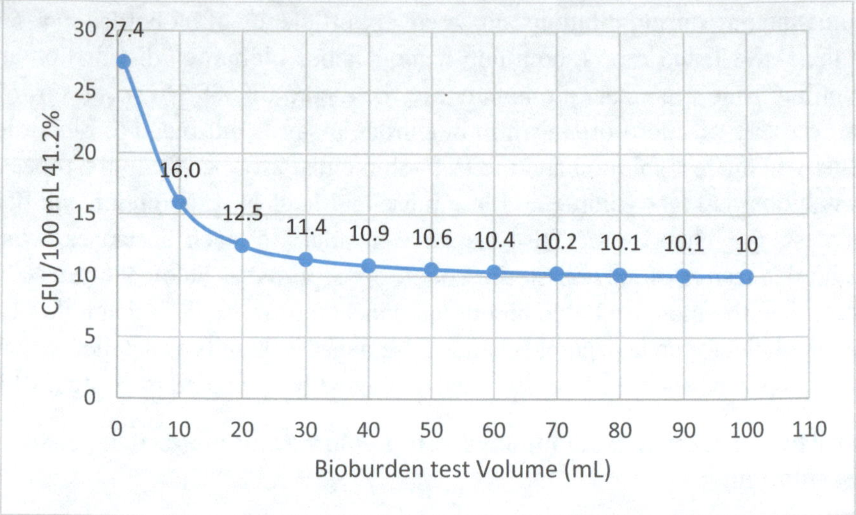

***Figure 1**: Minimum microbial load in a bioburden test volume with a sensitivity (41.2%) equal to that of a 100-mL test volume to detect 10 CFU.*

Step-2: Using the minimum bioburden concentration calculated for the sensitivity of 41.2% for the respective test volume as shown in Figure 1, one can also calculate the probability of false negative results at different bioburden concentration in test solutions at respective test volumes by applying negative binomial distribution model as shown equation-2 [4].

$$P_{false,neg} = 1 - NEGBINOM(F, S, p, True) \qquad \text{Eq. (2)}$$

Where,

$P_{\text{false, neg}}$ = probability of false negative results of bioburden test.

NEGBINOM: Returns the negative binomial distribution, the probability that there will be "F" failures before the "S" success, with "P_s" probability of a success.

F is the bioburden concentration in test solution ranging from 1 CFU/100mL

S is the $CFU/100mL_{41.2\%}$ is the minimum microbial load in a bioburden test volume with a sensitivity 41.2% for different bioburden test volume calculated using equation 1.

P_s probability of a success that is 41.2%.

Figure-2 shows the false negative probability of bioburden test at different test volume and bioburden concentration in test solution using equation 2.

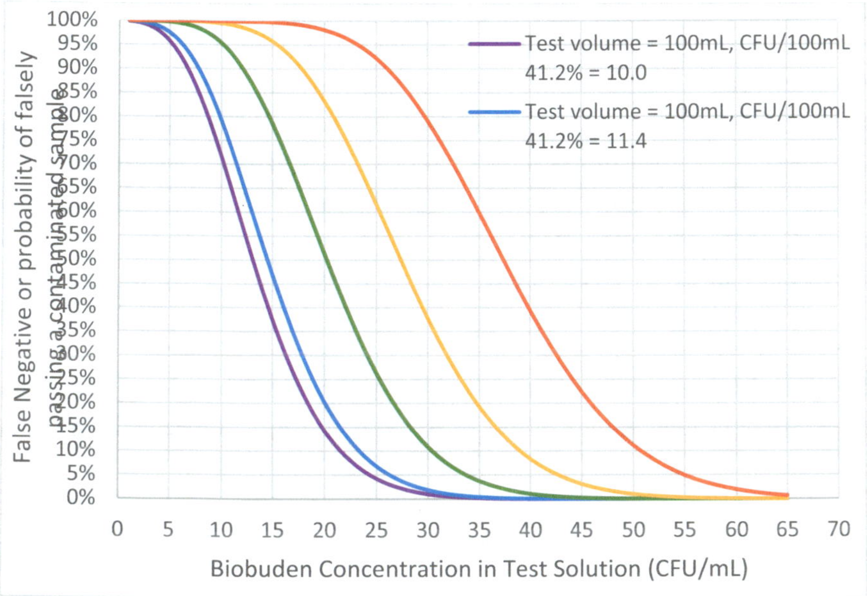

Figure 2: *False negative probability of bioburden test at different test volume and bioburden concentration in a test solution.*

From Figure 2 at an acceptable false negative risk of 0.05 on bioburden test result, for 1mL test volume, the bioburden concentration in the test solution is 55 CFU/100mL. This value is used as the initial bioburden load at the start of the medium preparation, X_0 in equation-3 to calculate the change in bioburden load over the hold period.

For any preparation the microbial risks are sourced from starting raw materials and Improperly cleaned or contaminated equipment. Assuming the media preparation is performed in a clean container and in a classified clean room, the major source of bioburden is from raw material. For formulation of typical chemically defined (CD) cell culture liquid media, approximately at least 95% of mass constitutes Water for Injection (WFI) and the remaining is constituted using dry powdered cell culture growth supplements [47]. For WFI, the maximum acceptable bioburden limit is 10 CFU/100mL per USP 29 <1231>, and for the dry powdered cell culture supplements, humidity at packing is $\leq 1\%$ to ensure stability [46], which is less than the humidity to promote any microbial growth (USP<1112> reported no microbial growth below water activity of 0.6, which is equivalent to humidity of 60%). Considering the formulated media constitutes 95% of WFI with maximum bioburden limit of 10 CFU/mL and the remaining of less than 5% of dry powdered supplement is micro-static in nature over short period from the time of dispensing to usage. A bioburden load of 55 CFU/100mL is a good conservative estimate for time (t=0).

Modeling Bioburden Proliferation during the Pre-Filtration Hold Time: The increase in bioburden load for different hold times is calculated by using Eq. 3 [5].

$$X_i = X_0 \times e^{(\Delta t \times \mu)} \qquad \text{Eq. (3)}$$

Here, X_0 is the microbial load at time t=0 as calculated from Eq. 1, X_i is the bioburden load at time t=i, and μ is the specific growth rate. The value of specific growth rate (μ) is heavily influenced by media preparation temperature. Often, most cell culture media are prepared at ambient room temperature (15°C to 25°C) to avoid nutrient degradation; therefore, a preparation temperature of 21°C is a good approximation. Rosso et al. (1993) gave a cardinal growth model to predict the Influence of temperature on microbial-specific growth rate, as shown in Eq.4 [16].

$$\mu = \frac{\mu_{max} \times (T - T_{min})^2 \times (T - T_{max})}{(T_{opt} - T_{min}) \times [(T_{opt} - T_{min}) \times (T - T_{opt}) - (T_{opt} - T_{max}) \times (T_{opt} + T_{min} - 2T)]} \quad \text{Eq. (4)}$$

Where,

μ_{max} is the maximum specific growth rate. As a conservative approach, the (μ_{max}) is assumed for *Escherichia coli*, one of the fastest-doubling bacterial species with the doubling time T_d of 20 min or 0.3 hr [17] from which the value of μ_{max} is calculated as 2.1 hr^{-1} using equation, μ_{max}= Ln(2)/T_d, where Ln(2) is natural logarithm of 2.

T_{min} and T_{max} are minimum and maximum temperatures, respectively, at which microbial growth is no longer observed and T_{opt} refers to optimum temperature for microbial growth. Rosson et al.(1993) showed for E.coli, T_{min} = 4.9°C, T_{opt}= 41.4°C, and T_{max}=45.8°C. [18]. Applying all the above assumptions and media preparation temperature T= 21°C, the calculated value for μ using Eq.3 is 0.5 hr^{-1} that can be substituted in Eq- 2 to calculate the change in microbial load over hold time.

Post-filtration Risk: The post-filtration risk is defined as the probability of having at least 1 CFU pass through the filtration system. This risk can be calculated via Eq. 5 [6]:

$$R_{pf} = 1 - (1 - p_1)^{(V_f \times X_i)} \quad \text{Eq. (5)}$$

Where, R_{pf} is the post-filtration risk. For upstream media and feed, any microbial breach is frequently identified by a reduction in pH and/or in the dissolved oxygen trend in the bioreactor early in the process, prior to the purification process, well before the batch is released. Therefore, based on the batch run rate, an R_{pf} value of 10^{-3} is well accepted in practice, indicating that only 1 out of 1,000 batches would have a microbial breakthrough during filtration. For a run rate of 10 batches in a 20,000-L production bioreactor per year, one batch per 100 years is an acceptable risk.

The term ($V_f \times X_i$) gives the total microbial load in the solution challenging the 0.22-μm filters ($mL/cm^2 \times CFU/mL = CFU/cm^2$). V_f is the filtrate throughput in mL/cm^2, and X_i is the bioburden load in CFU/mL. p_1 is the probability that one bacterium to successfully pass through filer membrane per cm^2, which follows a binomial distribution. p_1 can be derived from the binomial confidence interval, calculated as shown in Eq. 6 [6-7].

$$p_1 = \frac{F.DIST(\alpha, S+1, N)}{N + F.DIST(\alpha, S+1, N)} \qquad \text{Eq. (6)}$$

Here, F.Dist calculates the cumulative probability density function for the F Distribution in Microsoft Excel, Statistical confidence (1-α) is assumed to be 0.95 by default. Therefore, $\alpha = 0.05$ in Eq.6, S is the number of successful events. Here, the event is defined as to be number of bacteria to penetrate through the sterile filter area. Therefore, for one bacterium to breakthrough sterile filter area, the event (S) is assumed be =1, and N is the number of trials required for achieving at least one successful event; N is equal to maximum retention capacity of the filter obtained from filter manufacturers certificate of analysis (COA). In most cases, 0.22-μm sterile filters in the market are rated for a microbial retention capacity of 1E7 CFU per square centimeter based on bacterial species Brevundimonas diminuta.

In biologics manufacturing process, often pre-filtration is performed using 0.45 μm pore size membrane filters before 0.22 μm sterile filtration. Carter. J (1996) showed a bacterial retention capacity of 10^4 CFU/cm^2 using Pseudomonas diminuta for 0.45 μm pore size membrane filters [27], and PDA technical article No.26 reported the microbial penetration is observed through 0.45 μm pore size membrane filters when challenged with microbial load above 10^{-4} to

10^{-6} per cm^2 [28]. Therefore, conservatively maximum microbial retention capacity (N) for 0.45 µm pore size membrane filters is assumed to be 10^4 CFU/cm^2. In such prefiltration usage instances, the post-filtration risk is calculated independently for 0.45 µm and 0.22 µm pore size membrane filters using Eq-4 and then the risks for both 0.45 µm and 0.22 µm pore size membrane filters are multiplied to get the post filtration risk on combined set up of prefiltration followed by post filtration system.

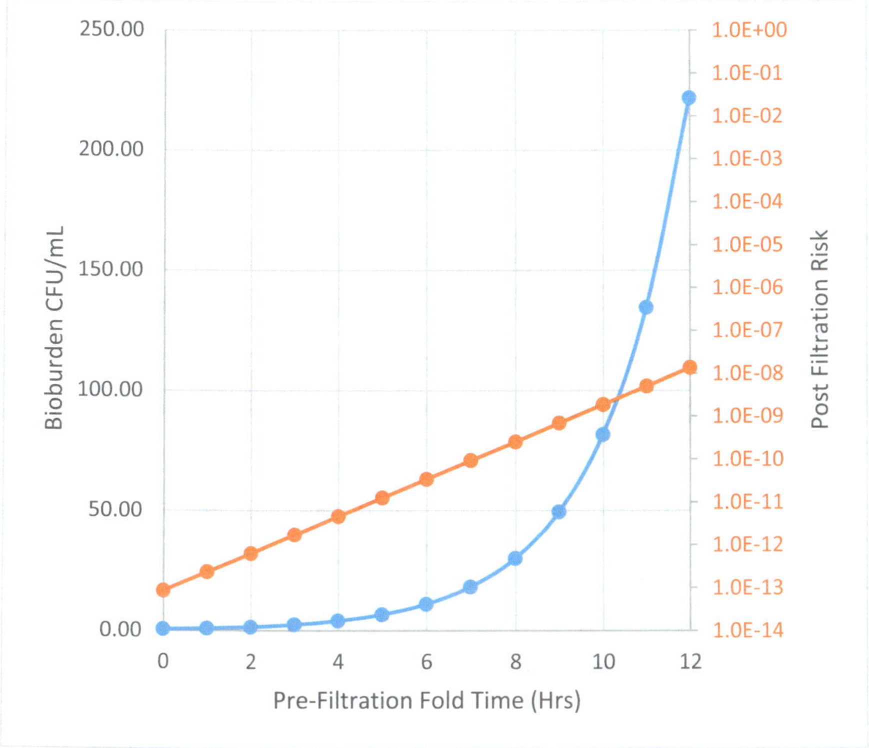

Figure 3: *Change in microbial load and post-filtration risk vs. pre-filtration hold time.*

Bioburden Acceptance Criteria Vs. Bioburden Load Challenge before Filtration: Sandle, T. (2022) reported that a maximum pre-sterilization bioburden limit of 1,000 CFU/mL is a suitable limit for the starting material or first stage of a manufacturing process [8]. As shown in Figure 1, the calculated bioburden load after a pre-filtration hold time of $4T_p$= 12 hours is 4.5 folds below the limit of 1,000 CFU/mL = 221 CFU/mL.

Risk based Approach for Calculating Pre-Filtration Bioburden Acceptance Criteria: Yang (2013) presented risk-based approach for calculating pre-filtration bioburden acceptance criteria, where post-filtration risk is set based on the risk assessment, then pre-filtration bioburden acceptance criteria is calculated as a function of filter area, filtrate volume and maximum retention capacity of the sterile filter that are specific to the process as shown in equation-7. Eq 7 is obtained by re-arranging terms in equation 4.

$$x_{Accp} \leq \left[\frac{\ln(1 - R_{pf})}{\ln(1 - P_1)}\right] \div V_f \qquad \text{Eq. (7)}$$

Box-1 shows the sample Calculation for setting pre-filtration Bioburden limit.

Box-1: Sample Calculation for setting pre-filtration Bioburden limit
Step 1: Calculate the Filtrate throughput in (mL/cm^2); for the purpose of illustration, media throughput (**V_f**) of 1000 L/m^2 equivalent to 100 mL/cm^2 is assumed. **Step 2:** Setting post-filtration risk (**R_{pf}**) based on risk assessment. Acceptable risks are wider in upstream processes and get tighter toward the end of the downstream processes. Using risk assessment matrix as shown in Table-1, for upstream media and feed pre-filtration, the risk is classified as low, and thereby, the post-filtration risk is selected as 1.0E-3. **Step 3:** Calculate the **(p1)** the probability that one bacterium will successfully pass through one cm^2 filter area. $$p_1 = \frac{F.DIST(0.05, (1+1), 1E7)}{N + F.DIST(0.05, (1+1), 1E7)} = 4.9 \times 10^{-09}$$ **Step 4:** Calculate the minimum acceptable bioburden limit.

Box-1: Sample Calculation for setting pre-filtration Bioburden limit
$x_{Accp} \leq \left[\frac{\ln(1-1\times10^{-3})}{\ln(1-4.9\times10^{-9})}\right] \div \left[100\,\frac{mL}{cm^2}\right] = 2{,}041$ CFU/mL
To mitigate any potential risk of microbial breach during sterile filtration, as a good design practice, sterile filters are often oversized and therefore, the calculated minimum bioburden acceptance criteria using this procedure is often going to be larger than the recommended 1000 CFU/mL by Sandle T (2022). Therefore, I advocate to conservatively use 1000 CFU/mL as acceptance criteria and verify the suitability of using 1000 CFU/mL by risk assessment using calculation as detailed in Box-1.

Table 1: Risk Assessment Matrix for Setting Post-Filtration Risk

Severity [s]	Occurrence [C]	Detectability [D]	Score	RPN =[S]×[C]× [D]	Risk Category	Post Filtration Risk R_{pf}
No product impact, Potential Impact to the process at early stage of the process before start of purification	Effective controls are in place at multiple subsequent unit operations to fully mitigate the risk	Microbial safety is tested as (In-process control) IPC more than once before moving forward into final DS formulation	1	1 to 25	Low	1.0E-03

Table 1: Risk Assessment Matrix for Setting Post-Filtration Risk

Severity [s]	**Occurrence [C]**	**Detectability [D]**	**Score**	**RPN =[S]×[C]×[D]**	**Risk Category**	**Post Filtration Risk R_{pf}**
No product Impact, Potential Impact to the process during purification.	Only limited one stage controls is there before sterile drug formulation. However, not comprehensive enough to fully mitigate the risk at high confidence	Microbial safety is tested as IPC only once before moving forward for final DS formulation	3	26 to 50	Medium	1.0E-04
Potential to impact product safety at DS/DP stage	No controls are in place	Microbial safety is tested only on formulated DS/DP	5	≥ 51	High	1.0E-06 (1)

(1) The sterility assurance level (SAL): A SAL of 10-6 means that there is less than or equal to one chance in a million that a single viable microorganism is present on a sterilized item [32].
(2)

The minimum acceptable pre-filtration bioburden limit calculated in (CFU/mL) using Eq.7 is plotted against the filtrate throughput (L/cm^2) for different post filtration risk is shown in Figure 4, which can be used as a handy tool.

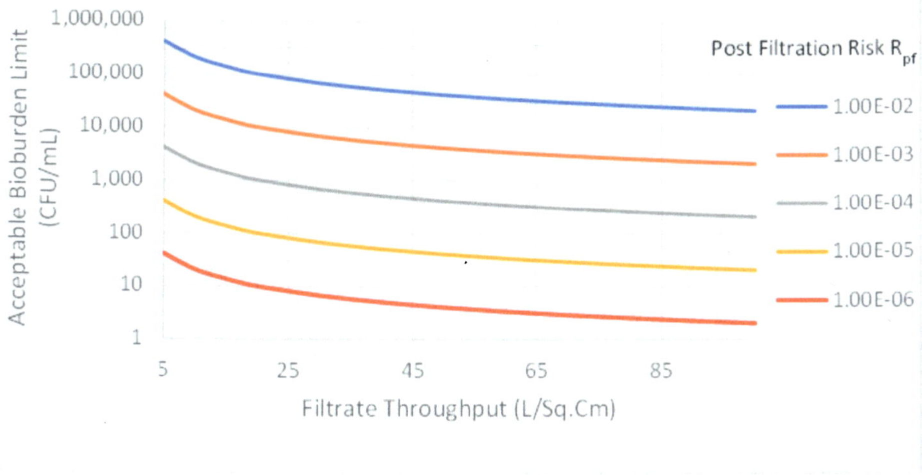

Figure 4: *Minimum acceptable pre-filtration bioburden limit in (CFU/mL) V.s the filtrate throughput (L/cm2) at different post-filtration risk*

Change in Exotoxin Load and Clearance in Downstream: Although a bioburden can be easily removed by 0.22-µm filtration, residual microbial by-products may be co-purified with the product and may have detrimental effects on patient safety and product quality. Microbial by-products that can have adverse effects on patient safety primarily include protein exotoxins (e.g., botulinum toxin A), non-protein exotoxins (e.g., aflatoxin, endotoxins, flagellin, microbial DNA, and cell wall polysaccharides). With the exception of endotoxins, there are no available good manufacturing practice (GMP) assays for detecting these microbial by-products. However, levels of exotoxin components can be calculated and compared with safety levels using worst-case assumptions [9].

The in-product impurity dose of produced exotoxin can be conservatively calculated as shown in Eq. 8. Botulinum toxin-A is an exotoxin that presents safety concerns even at very low doses compared with other exotoxins. Therefore, botulinum A is used as the worst-case representation of all other exotoxins [11, 12].

$$IDP_{Exo} = \Sigma x_i \frac{CFU}{mL} \times Y_{Protein/cell} \frac{pg\ of\ protein}{CFU} \times 0.05\% \times DP \frac{mL}{Kg} \qquad \text{Eq. (8)}$$

Here, IDP_{Exo} is the in-product impurity dose for exotoxin (pg/kg), ΣX_i (CFU/mL) is the cumulative amount of microbial load produced until time t=i (Refer Figure:5 for details for calculation), Protein yield per microbial cell $Y_{protein/Cell}$ is assumed to be 0.165 pg of protein/microbial cell [19]. Wintzingerode, F. V. (2017) cited 0.05% of the bacterial protein mass as protein exotoxins. As a conservative approach, all the total protein exotoxins calculated are considered as Botulinum-A [12].

The typical range of protein concentration in formulated drug product ranges from 50 and 150 mg/ml for monoclonal antibodies (mAbs) [20], with dosing quantity going as high as 10 mg/kg of patient weight [21]. DP is the drug product dose in mL/kg (for the purpose of illustration, DP dose is conservatively calculated as 10 mg/Kg ÷ 50 mg/mL= 0.2 mL/kg of patient body weight).

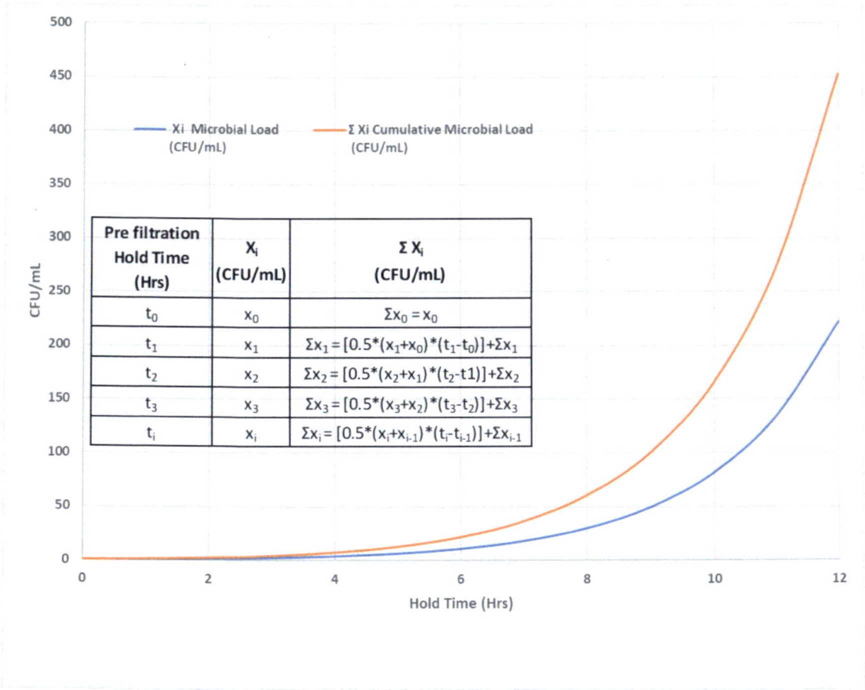

Pre filtration Hold Time (Hrs)	X_i (CFU/mL)	ΣX_i (CFU/mL)
t_0	x_0	$\Sigma x_0 = x_0$
t_1	x_1	$\Sigma x_1 = [0.5*(x_1+x_0)*(t_1-t_0)]+\Sigma x_1$
t_2	x_2	$\Sigma x_2 = [0.5*(x_2+x_1)*(t_2-t1)]+\Sigma x_2$
t_3	x_3	$\Sigma x_3 = [0.5*(x_3+x_2)*(t_3-t_2)]+\Sigma x_3$
t_i	x_i	$\Sigma x_i = [0.5*(x_i+x_{i-1})*(t_i-t_{i-1})]+\Sigma x_{i-1}$

Figure 5: *ΣX_i is the cumulative amount of microbial load produced until time t= i (CFU/mL)*

Exotoxin Clearance Across Protein A Chromatography: In biologics manufacturing processes, protein A affinity chromatography is typically the first step in purification. The interaction between IgG and protein A has been shown to be highly specific, and this affinity mode of chromatography enables the removal of >99% of process impurities in a single step, starting directly from complex solutions such as cell culture clarified harvest media [23]. Therefore, both exotoxins and endotoxins should be substantially cleared by a protein affinity column process. An exotoxin spike study demonstrated a 1.9 log reduction value (LRV) or 98.7% clearance over MabSelect SuRe [13]. Thus, as a conservative approach, an LRV of 1 may be used for exotoxin clearance calculations.

Exotoxin Clearance Across Cation Exchange (CEx) Chromatography: The net protein surface charge changes with the pH of the buffer based on the iso-electric point (PI). At a pH equal to the PI, the protein will carry no net charge. At a pH below the PI, the protein attains a net positive charge; similarly, at a pH above the PI, the protein will attain a net negative charge.

The CEx step is performed in a bind/elute mode. Typically, the buffer has a pH of 4–6, which is below the PI (>7) of most monoclonal antibodies (mAbs). At a buffer pH between 4 and 6, the mAb attains a positive charge, allowing it to bind negatively charged resin. The PI for exotoxins is approximately 2.5. Therefore, exotoxin impurities attain a negative charge and will flow through the chromatography column; thus, the exotoxins should be greatly cleared by the CEx step of the process. An exotoxin spike study showed an LRV of 2.9 in clearance over CEx chromatography [13]. Thus, as a conservative approach, an LRV of 3 may be used for exotoxin clearance calculations across overall purification process.

Change in Endotoxin Load: Endotoxin A is a pyrogenic product present in the bacterial cell wall, which can lead to adverse reactions ranging from fever to death in a patient, even at a trace concentration of 0.1 ng per kg patient body weight. Thus, endotoxins present another risk associated with the microbial load that arises when process intermediates are held. Liposaccharide or endotoxin is produced at 10^{-15} g per gram of typical negative bacterium. Endotoxins are reported in endotoxin units (EU), where 0.1 ng is equal to 1 EU [15]. The in-product impurity dose for endotoxins during the pre-filtration medium hold time is calculated as shown in Eq. 9

$$IDP_{endo} = \Sigma X_i \frac{CFU}{mL} \times \frac{10^{-06} ng\ of\ Endotoxin}{CFU} \times DP \frac{mL}{Kg} \qquad \text{Eq. (9)}$$

Endotoxin Clearance Across anion exchange (AEx) chromatography: In anion exchange (AEx) chromatography, the protein of interest is recovered in the flow-through mode. In AEx, under neutral or slightly basic pH conditions, endotoxins are negatively charged and bind tightly to positively charged resin and target protein flowing through the column. Additional information on endotoxin clearance is detailed in Box-2.

Endotoxin Acceptance Criteria: Acceptable limits for endotoxins can be wider in upstream processes and tighter toward the end of the downstream processes based on the understanding of process risk and endotoxin clearance capabilities. Endotoxin limits for in-process intermediates are determined based on the clearance factor, the total potential for introduction of endotoxin to the product and quantitation limit.

The quantification limits and acceptable endotoxin limit are calculated based on worst-case assay dilution and protein concentration in formulated drug substance (DS), as shown in Box-2.

Box-2: Sample Calculation for setting pre-filtration Endotoxin limit [14, 25]

Step-1: Maximum Valid Dilution (MVD) is calculated as a function of sensitivity of the assay technique used, acceptable level of endotoxin in patient dose based on route of administration, maximum product dose, and patient population.

- λ is sensitivity of the assay (EU/mL). Though, different techniques like Gel-Clot Technique, Turbidimetric Technique or Chromo-clots the lysate are available. The type of endotoxin detection assay used depends on the product and dilution required to overcome inhibition and enhancement as per USP <85>. For the purpose of illustration, sensitivity (λ) =0.005 for Turbidimetric Technique is used.
- **AL_{Endo}**: Per USP<85> Acceptable limit of endotoxin is 5 EU/kg of body weight for any route of administration other than intrathecal (for which it is 0.2 EU/kg of body weight). As a conservative approach, we assume AL_{Endo} = 0.2 EU/Kg.
- **C_{DP},** protein concentration in formulated drug product, conservatively assumed to be at 50 mg/mL from a published range of 50 to 100 mg/L [20].
- **M** is equal to the maximum recommended bolus dose of product per kg of body weight based on dose, drug type, and population weight as referenced USP <85>. For the purpose of illustration, M is conservatively assumed to be 10 mg/Kg [21].

Box-2: Sample Calculation for setting pre-filtration Endotoxin limit [14, 25]

$$MVD = \frac{\left[AL_{Endo}\,\frac{EU}{kg} \div M\,\frac{mg}{kg}\right] \times C_{DP}\,\frac{mg}{mL}}{\lambda\,\frac{EU}{mL}} = \frac{\left[0.2\,\frac{EU}{kg} \div 10\,\frac{mg}{kg}\right] \times 50\,\frac{mg}{mL}}{0.005\,\frac{EU}{mL}}$$

$$= 200$$

Step-2: Quantification Limit (QL) for worst case Dilution factor and Protein Concentration is calculated as:

$$QL = \lambda \times \frac{MVD}{C_{DP}} = 0.005\,\frac{EU}{mL} \times \frac{200}{50\,\frac{mg}{mL}} = 0.02\,\frac{EU}{mg}$$

Step-3: Acceptable Endotoxin Limit is calculated based on the QL and clearance factor in purification (CFp) as follows:

$$AL_{Endo} = \left[QL\,\frac{EU}{mg} \times C_{DP}\,\frac{mg}{mL}\right] \div \left[CF_p \times V_f \times k\right]$$

- Banerjee S (2012) presented Endotoxin clearance from 0.9 LRV to 3.0 LRV across four different AEx resins at different buffer conditions, additionally up to 4 LRV clearance has been shown using charged Durapore® 0.22 µm filters and another 4 LRV reduction using ultrafiltration membrane sizes ranging from 10-1000 KD [26]. However, Magalhães P (2007) indicates in the pharmaceutical industry, diversity among endotoxins based on the source of micro-organisms there is a dilemma in their effective removal from the process stream. As all the above-cited endotoxin clearance are based on spike studies using specific types of endotoxins, as a conservative approach for the purpose of illustration overall clearance **CFp** = 2.0 LRV or 0.01 factor is selected. Readers should evaluate the selected endotoxin clearance specific to their process.
- The Limulus amebocyte lysate (LAL) endotoxin test is an enzyme-based assay, incur with expected 2-fold inherent variability as reported by Sandle T (2014) [29,30]. Therefore, $\mathbf{V_f}$ is assumed to be 2.0.
- **K** = 3 is the common statistical tolerance factor used to represent 99.7% of the population (e.g. ± 3×SD (Standard deviation)). This approach of including 3 × V_f in setting endotoxin limits is used by Wintzingerode, F (2017).

Box-2: Sample Calculation for setting pre-filtration Endotoxin limit [14, 25]
$$AL_{Endo} = \left[0.02\ \frac{EU}{mg} \times 50 \frac{mg}{mL}\right] \div [0.01 \times 2 \times 3] = 16\ \frac{EU}{mL}$$ **Note:** Though different cell lines are sensitive to different levels of endotoxin from 0.1 to 10 ng/mL, cell lines like CHO, HeLa and Murine cells that have been cultured for protein production have been naturally selected for high endotoxin resistance by long-term inadvertent exposure of endotoxin sourced from growth media and sera [33]. The lowest concentration of endotoxin that is shown to affect the recombinant CHO and Murine cell protein production is 10 ng/mL, equivalent to 100 EU/mL [34, 35]. When no historic data is available for pre-filtration upstream media and feed solution, I advocate to conservatively use the lowest reported endotoxin level to impact the cell culture; that is 0.1 ng/mL, equivalent to 10EU/mL as provisional endotoxin limits to start with, which is within the calculated endotoxin safety limits based on extreme worst-case assumptions as shown in this Box-2. Later as more data is available and knowledge in microbial control with facility set-up is matured, the limits can be narrowed down further.

Impurity Safety Factor (ISF) Risk Assessment for Exotoxins and Endotoxins: Safety risk assessments can be carried out via ISF calculations. The ISF is the ratio of the impurity level in the product to the toxic impurity level. The ISF can be calculated as shown in Eq. 10 [10].

$$ISF = \frac{TD_{Lo}}{Impurity\ Level\ in\ Product\ (IDP)} \qquad \text{Eq. (10)}$$

Toxic dose low (TD_{Lo}): The lowest dose of a substance introduced by any route, other than inhalation, over any given period of time and reported to produce any toxic effect in humans or to produce tumorigenic or reproductive effects in animals. A higher ISF indicates a lower safety risk.

Here, we assume the Toxic dose low (TD_{Lo}) for botulinum A to be 1.2 pg per kg of patient weight per hour [11]. For Endotoxin, the lowest FDA-recommended dose for is 0.2 EU per kg of body weight per hour for intrathecally administered products. Assuming 1 EU = 0.1ng, (TD_{Lo}) value for endotoxin is assumed to be 0.02 ng per kg of body weight per hour [22,24].

Figure 6 shows after considering 3LRV clearance of exotoxin and 2 LRV clearance of endotoxin in downstream processes, the calculated exotoxin and endotoxin ISF values are 100,000 and 10,000 times below the toxic dose.

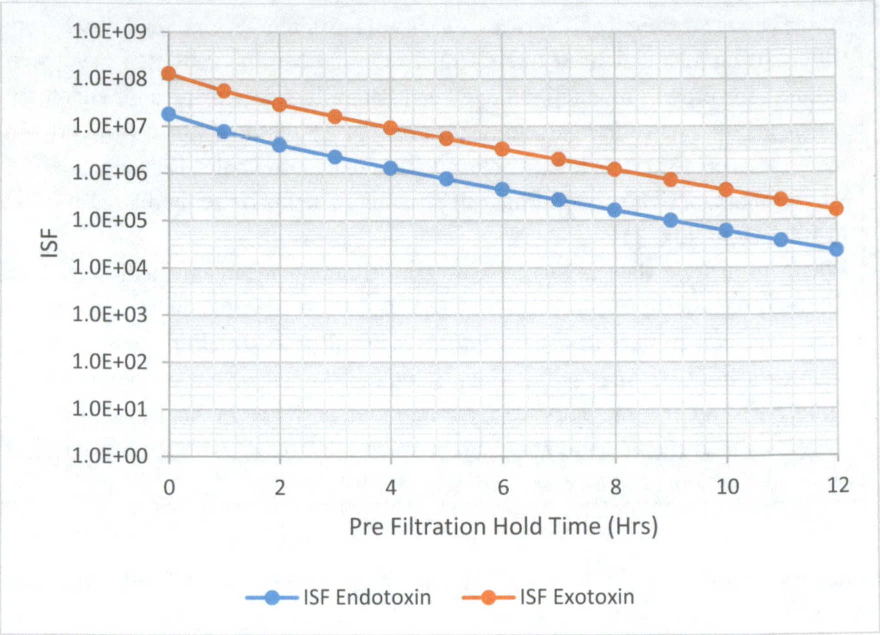

***Figure 6**: ISF for endotoxins and exotoxins vs. pre-filtration hold time.*

Bioburden and Endotoxin Criteria for Routine and other process validation samples:

As the risk assessment for bioburden and endotoxin calculations in Box-1 and Box-2, respectively, may be applied for setting bioburden and endotoxin acceptance criteria for other upstream routine manufacturing and process validation samples. As an extended scope from the pre-filtration microbial control focus, Table-2, details on guidance and rational for alert and action limits for routine manufacturing and process validation upstream samples.

Sample Type	Upstream Unit Operation	Sample Description	Reg. Req.	Bioburden (CFU/mL)	Endotoxin (EU/mL)
R	Cell Expansion	Testing for bioburden of the final culture vessel from passive control inoculum expansion (Cultibag) to the first active control expansion may be tested or kept as a back-up sample (perform a purity check under microscope in the case of microbial processes).	No [11]	Alert: 1 CFU/10mL (A) Action: 10 CFU/10mL (B)	Not Required
R	Seed Bioreactor	Prior to transfer into the next bioreactor, a bioburden sample may be tested or kept as a backup sample (perform a purity check under microscope in the case of microbial processes).	No [11]	Alert: 1 CFU/10mL (A) Action: 10 CFU/10mL (B)	Not Required
RS	Production Bioreactor	In the case of production bioreactors, all batches should be tested for bioburden at the end of production (unprocessed bulk sample). Endotoxin testing is not routinely performed at inoculum expansion stages since these stages are expected to be essentially sterile.	Yes [37]	Alert: > 1 CFU/10mL (A) Action:>10 CFU/10mL (B)	Alert: > 5 EU/mL [C] Action: > 10 EU/mL [D]
RS	Harvest	Clarified harvest pool (0.22 μm filtered) at the end of harvest operations should be tested for bioburden/endotoxin for all batches just prior to the start of the following process step.	Yes [38]	Alert: 1 CFU/10mL (A) Action: 10 CFU/10mL (B)	Alert: > 5 EU/mL [C] Action: > 10 EU/mL [D]

Sample Type	Upstream Unit Operation	Sample Description	Reg. Req.	Bioburden (CFU/mL)	Endotoxin (EU/mL)
PV	Media, Feed Prep / Filtration	Pre-filtration sample for upstream growth media and Feeds	Yes: [39]	Alert: >200 CFU/mL [E] Action:>1000 CFU/mL [F]	Alert: > 5 EU/mL [C] Action: > 10 EU/mL [D]
PV	Filtered Media Storage in Sterile container	Post filtration media storage for up to 24 hours at 2-8°C or up to 12 hours at room temperature 19 to 25°C in sterile storage tanks/ bags/bioreactors. [40,41]		Alert: 1 CFU/10mL (A) Action: 10 CFU/10mL (B)	Alert: > 5 EU/mL [C] Action: > 10 EU/mL [D]
PV	Production Bioreactor	LIVCA (Limit of Invitro Cell Age)	Yes: [42],[43]	Alert: 1 CFU/10mL (A) Action: 10 CFU/10mL (B)	Not Required
PV	Harvest	Equilibration and Chase buffer storage for up to 24 hours at 2-8°C or up to 12 hours at room temperature 19 to 25°C in sterile storage tanks/ bags before use. [40,41]	Yes [39]	Alert: 1 CFU/10mL (A) Action: 10 CFU/10mL (B)	Alert: > 5 EU/mL [C] Action: > 10 EU/mL [D]

RS: Routine sample
PV: Process validation sample
Reg. Req: Regulatory requirement
[A] No microbial growth expected in sterile sample from bioreactor.
[B] Deutschmann, S., & Thoelken, S. (2022) cited for BDS samples taken aseptically from Class D, C and B and analyzed in a non-classified microbiological laboratory, a couple of colonies can appear on plates from sampling or handling. This may cause occasional false positive results (Falsely rejecting a batch) [44]. In such instances, setting bioburden an action limit of 10 CFU/10mL in addition to the alert limit of 1CFU/10mL as recommended by Krause S (2015) [14] May be adopted as an acceptable limit to avoid Falsely rejecting a good batch.
[C] As discussed in endotoxin clearance section, one of the most effective purification steps used in downstream for endotoxin removal is anion-exchange chromatography (A_{EX}). FDA cited an IPC limit of 5 EU/mL for Anion exchange product pool in downstream for mAb production process [45]. Therefore, setting 5 EU/mL as provisional alert limits early in the manufacturing process (for upstream media and feed solutions) should be a good acceptable approach.
[D] Based on the calculation in Box-2.
[E] Based microbial load change data shown in Figure-1.
[F] Based on calculation in Box-1.

Conclusions

In summary, this report has shown that bioburden and endotoxin test results meet the acceptable criteria for an extended pre-filtration hold time of $4T_p = 12$ hrs for 20,000L medium preparation. A conservative calculation was applied to model the change in bioburden load, risk of filtration failure, and ISF for exotoxins and endotoxins. The results demonstrated that the risk associated with microbial control during the pre-filtration hold time of 12 hours is well within acceptable risk limits. The risk assessments and calculations for microbial limits shown in this article are only for demonstration of procedures. The readers are highly encouraged to assess the suitability of acceptability of risks in adherence to the company's quality policy. Furthermore, the bioburden and endotoxin limits cited or calculated in this article may be used as provisional limits when no historic data or only limited data is available. I highly recommend that the provisional limits are re-evaluated based on generated data.

References

1. [1] FDA. (2020, May 4). Sterile drug products produced by aseptic processing — Current good. https://www.fda.gov/regulatory-information/search-fda-guidance-documents/sterile-drug-products-produced-aseptic-processing-current-good-manufacturing-practice
2. [2] General Chapter <1115> Bioburden Control for Non-Sterile Drug Substance and Products. USP 41; U.S. Pharmacopeia 2014
3. [3] Sandle, T. (2015, October). Assessing Process Hold Times for Microbial Risks: Bioburden and Endotoxin. Journal of GXP Compliance, 19(3).
4. [4] Yang, H., Li, N., & Chang, S. (2013). A risk-based approach to setting sterile filtration Bioburden limits. PDA Journal of Pharmaceutical Science and Technology, 67(6), 601-609. https://doi.org/10.5731/pdajpst.2013.00942
5. [5] Doran, P. M. (2013). Bioprocess engineering principles. Academic Press.
6. [6] Coffey, T., & Yang, H. (2018). Statistics for biotechnology process development. CRC Press.
7. [7] Muralidharan, N. (2022, October). Statistical Method for Establishing Control Limits for Nonnormal Data Distribution: Focus on Continued Process Verification Monitoring. Bioprocess International, 20(10), 20-24.
8. [8] Sandle, T. (2022, October 1). What Counts? Establishing a Bioburden Strategy for a New Pharmaceutical Product. American Pharmaceutical Review.
9. [9] Sandle, T. (2014, November 28). The Risk of Bacillus cereus to Pharmaceutical Manufacturing. American Pharmaceutical Review. https://www.americanpharmaceuticalreview.com/Featured-Articles/169507-The-Risk-of-em-Bacillus-cereus-em-to-Pharmaceutical-Manufacturing/
10. [10] Luo, H., Li, Y., Robbins, D., Wang, S., Xi, G., Cox, M., Nicholson, S. M., Wei, C., Pabst, T. M., & Wang, W. K. (2021). Safety risk management for low molecular weight process-related impurities in monoclonal antibody therapeutics: Categorization, risk assessment, testing strategy, and process development with leveraging clearance

potential. Biotechnology Progress, 37(3). https://doi.org/10.1002/btpr.3119

11. [11] Bain, D., Hardy, D., Bell, B. L., Forng, R., Knight, M., Bawa, A., Ramsey, S., Arbesser-Rastburg, C., Paul, M., Ton, C., Leira, F., Roman, C., McFarland, K., Phillips, D., Stuckey, J., Bauer, C., & Calvo, A. J. (2015). Microbial monitoring for biological drug substance manufacturing: An industry perspective. PDA Journal of Pharmaceutical Science and Technology, 69(3), 451-460. https://doi.org/10.5731/pdajpst.2015.01070
12. [12] Wintzingerode, F. V. (2017, April 30). Biologics Production: Impact of Bioburden Contaminations of Non-Sterile Process Intermediates on Patient Safety and Product Quality. American Pharmaceutical Review. https://www.americanpharmaceuticalreview.com/Featured-Articles/337286-Biologics-Production-Impact-of-Bioburden-Contaminations-of-Non-Sterile-Process-Intermediates-on-Patient-Safety-and-Product-Quality/
13. [13] Cytiva. (2020). Exotoxin clearance from mAb samples in a two-step chromatography process (KA1638100118AN). https://cdn.cytivalifesciences.com/api/public/content/digi-24162-pdf
14. [14] Krause, S. (2015, March). Alert, Action, and Specification Limits for Bioburden and Endotoxin [Conference session]. PDA Annual Meeting, Las Vegas, NV.
15. [15] Salema, V. F., Saxena, L., & Pattnaik, P. (2009, September 30). Removing endotoxin from biopharmaceutical solutions. Pharmaceutical Technology Europe, 21(10), 16-20.
16. [16] Baka, M., Van Derlinden, E., Boons, K., Mertens, L., & Van Impe, J. F. (2013). Impact of pH on the cardinal temperatures of E. coli K12: Evaluation of the gamma hypothesis. Food Control, 29(2), 328-335. https://doi.org/10.1016/j.foodcont.2012.04.022
17. [17] Tuttle, A. R., Trahan, N. D., & Son, M. S. (2021). Growth and Maintenance of Escherichia coli Laboratory Strains. Current protocols, 1(1), e20. https://doi.org/10.1002/cpz1.20
18. [18] Membré, J. M., Leporq, B., Vialette, M., Mettler, E., Perrier, L., Thuault, D., & Zwietering, M. (2005). Temperature effect on bacterial growth rate: quantitative microbiology approach including cardinal values

and variability estimates to perform growth simulations on/in food. International journal of food microbiology, 100(1-3), 179–186. https://doi.org/10.1016/j.ijfoodmicro.2004.10.015

19. [19] Milo, R., & Phillips, R. (2015). Cell biology by the numbers. Garland Science.
20. [20] Garidel, P., Kuhn, A. B., Schäfer, L. V., Karow-Zwick, A. R., & Blech, M. (2017). High-concentration protein formulations: How high is high? European Journal of Pharmaceutics and Biopharmaceutics, 119, 353-360. https://doi.org/10.1016/j.ejpb.2017.06.029
21. [21] Sachs, J. R., Mayawala, K., Gadamsetty, S., Kang, S. P., & de Alwis, D. P. (2016). Optimal Dosing for Targeted Therapies in Oncology: Drug Development Cases Leading by Example. Clinical cancer research : an official journal of the American Association for Cancer Research, 22(6), 1318–1324. https://doi.org/10.1158/1078-0432.CCR-15-1295
22. [22] EMD Millipore. (n.d.). Endotoxin Removal The Solution With Membrane Separation Technology Application Note. White Paper. https://www.sigmaaldrich.com/deepweb/assets/sigmaaldrich/product/documents/219/983/tb2999en-ms.pdf
23. [23] Mehta, K., Soderquist, R., Shah, P., Marchand, N., & Bolton, G. (2018, February 16). Comparing Performance of New Protein A Resins for Monoclonal Antibody Purification. American Pharmaceutical Review. https://www.americanpharmaceuticalreview.com/Featured-Articles/347357-Comparing-Performance-of-New-Protein-A-Resins-for-Monoclonal-Antibody-Purification/
24. [24] Food and Drug Administration (FDA). (2020). Setting Endotoxin Limits During Development of Investigational Oncology Drugs and Biological Products. Center for Drug Evaluation and Research. https://www.fda.gov/media/140410/download
25. [25] General Chapter <85> Bacterial Endotoxins Test.; U.S. Pharmacopeia 2012.
26. [26] Banerjee, S., & Somasundaram, G. (2012). Endotoxin Control and Clearance in Biomanufacturing. Millipore Sigma. https://www.sigmaaldrich.com/US/en/collections/webinars/endotoxin-control-and-clearance-in-biomanufacturing

27. [27] Carter J. (1996). Evaluation of recovery filters for use in bacterial retention testing of sterilizing-grade filters. PDA journal of pharmaceutical science and technology, 50(3), 147–153.
28. [28] PDA technical Report No.26, (TR 26) Revised 2008. Sterilizing Filtration of Liquids. (2008). pda journal of pharmaceutical science and technology.
29. [29] Sandle, T. (2014, August 28). Variability and Test Error with the LAL Assay. American Pharmaceutical Review. https://www.americanpharmaceuticalreview.com/Featured-Articles/167404-Variability-and-Test-Error-with-the-LAL-Assay/
30. [30] Wintzingerode, F. (2017). Setting Endotoxin In-Process Controls for Recombinant Therapeutic Proteins. American Pharmaceutical Review, 20-23. https://www.acciusa.com/pdfs/supplements/Endotoxin%20Detection%20Part%20V/Setting_Endotoxin_In_Process.pdf
31. [31] Magalhães, P. O., Lopes, A. M., Mazzola, P. G., Rangel-Yagui, C., Penna, T. C., & Pessoa, A., Jr (2007). Methods of endotoxin removal from biological preparations: a review. Journal of pharmacy & pharmaceutical sciences : a publication of the Canadian Society for Pharmaceutical Sciences, Societe canadienne des sciences pharmaceutiques, 10(3), 388–404.
32. [32] ANSI/AAMI ST79:2017/(R)2022; COMPREHENSIVE GUIDE TO STEAM STERILIZATION AND STERILITY ASSURANCE IN HEALTH CARE FACILITIES . (2017). AAMI.
33. [33] Corning. (2020, June). Endotoxins and Cell Culture. www.corning.com/lifesciences . https://www.corning.com/catalog/cls/documents/application-notes/TC-305.pdf
34. [34] Epstein, J., Kelly, C. E., Lee, M. M., & Donahoe, P. K. (1990). Effect of E. Coli endotoxin on mammalian cell growth and recombinant protein production. In Vitro Cellular & Developmental Biology, 26(12), 1121-1122. https://doi.org/10.1007/bf02623686
35. [35] Sibley, C. H., Terry, A., & Raetz, C. R. (1988). Induction of kappa light chain synthesis in 70Z/3 B lymphoma cells by chemically defined lipid a precursors. Journal of Biological Chemistry, 263(11), 5098-5103. https://doi.org/10.1016/s0021-9258(18)60684-2

36. [36] Field, R. (2013, May). Bioburden Control at the Sterile Filtration Step: A risk-based approach [Conference session]. European Biopharmaceutical Enterprises. https://docplayer.net/49110306-Bioburden-control-at-the-sterile-filtration-step-a-risk-based-approach.html
37. [37] ICH. (1997). ICH Topic Q 5 A (R1) Quality of Biotechnological Products: Viral Safety Evaluation of Biotechnology Products Derived from Cell Lines of Human or Animal Origin (CPMP/ICH/295/95). https://www.ema.europa.eu/en/documents/scientific-guideline/ich-q-5-r1-viral-safety-evaluation-biotechnology-products-derived-cell-lines-human-animal-origin_en.pdf
38. [38] FDA. (2021). CHAPTER 56—DRUG QUALITY ASSURANCE. https://www.fda.gov/media/75208/download
39. [39] FDA. (2004). Guidance for Industry Sterile Drug Products Produced by Aseptic Processing — Current Good Manufacturing Practice. https://www.fda.gov/media/71026/download
40. [40] EMA. (2017). Guideline on manufacture of the finished dosage form (EMA/CHMP/QWP/245074/2015). https://www.ema.europa.eu/en/documents/scientific-guideline/guideline-manufacture-finished-dosage-form-revision-1_en.pdf
41. [41] Broughton. (n.d.). Aseptic Processing of Biological Products: Current Regulatory Issues "Facing the Challenges of Drug Product Manufacturing". FDA. https://www.fda.gov/files/drugs/published/Aseptic-Processing-of-Biological-Products--Current-Regulatory-Issues--Candace-Gomez-Broughton--PhD.pdf
42. [42] European Medicines Agency. (1996). ICH Topic Q 5 B Quality of Biotechnological Products: Analysis of the Expression Construct in Cell Lines Used for Production of r-DNA Derived Protein Products. https://www.ema.europa.eu/en/documents/scientific-guideline/ich-q-5-b-analysis-expression-construct-cell-lines-used-production-r-dna-derived-protein-products_en.pdf
43. [43] Agalloco, J., DeSantis, P., Grilli, A., & Pavell, A. (2021). Handbook of validation in pharmaceutical processes (4th ed.). CRC Press.
44. [44] Deutschmann, S., & Thoelken, S. (2022, July 29). Bioburden - Regulatory Expectations and Practical Experiences. GMP Journal.

https://www.gmp-journal.com/current-articles/details/q-a-from-european-gmp-conference-bioburden-regulatory-expectations-and-practical-experiences.html

45. [45] FDA. (2021). Q12 Technical and Regulatory Considerations for Pharmaceutical Product Lifecycle Management Annexes Guidance for Industry. https://www.fda.gov/media/148477/download
46. [46] BioPlan Associates, Inc. (2014). Powder Culture Media Packaging, Preparation and Market Trends. www.thermofisher.com. https://assets.thermofisher.com/TFS-Assets/LSG/brochures/PowderMediaWhitePaper_LifeTech_Jan2014.pdf
47. [47] Gibco. (2018, June). CD CHO Medium User Guide. thermofisher.com. https://assets.thermofisher.com/TFS-Assets/LSG/manuals/MAN0007311_CD_CHO_Medium_UG.pdf

Contributors and Co-Authors

Emma Bolduc

MSAT Engineer

AGC Biologics, Boulder, CO USA

Tyler Younger

MSAT Engineer

AGC Biologics, Boulder, CO USA

Grace Chan

MSAT Engineer

AGC Biologics, Boulder, CO USA

Leyla Saeednia Rose, PhD

MSAT Senior Manager,

AGC Biologics, Boulder, CO USA

Mark Davis

Director, Quality Control

AGC Biologics, Boulder, CO USA

Alexander Elkin

Manufacturing Engineer

AGC Biologics, Boulder, CO USA

Made in the USA
Monee, IL
14 June 2026

54081208R00109